THE
EVERYTHING
POST WEIGHT LOSS SURGERY COOKBOOK

Dear Reader,

I felt compelled to write a book about life after weight loss surgery because there is so much misinformation being touted as fact in the media, on the Internet, and even in medical facilities. Patients who try to do research are often finding half-truths and outright incorrect information. I felt it was important to create a resource for patients that could be trusted.

I hope this book will make your life easier, helping you find your way through the many changes you will face in the months and years after your procedure.

This book is designed to help you with many aspects of your weight loss journey, including complications that require calling your surgeon, how to cook flavorful low-fat foods, varying your wardrobe, and even how to shop for groceries.

Enjoy the amazing journey that starts after weight loss surgery! There are countless changes ahead, many of which will be cause for celebration.

Jennifer Whitlock Heisler

Welcome to the EVERYTHING® Series!

These handy, accessible books give you all you need to tackle a difficult project, gain a new hobby, comprehend a fascinating topic, prepare for an exam, or even brush up on something you learned back in school but have since forgotten.

You can choose to read an *Everything*® book from cover to cover or just pick out the information you want from our four useful boxes: e-questions, e-facts, e-alerts, and e-ssentials.

We give you everything you need to know on the subject, but throw in a lot of fun stuff along the way, too.

We now have more than 400 *Everything*® books in print, spanning such wide-ranging categories as weddings, pregnancy, cooking, music instruction, foreign language, crafts, pets, New Age, and so much more. When you're done reading them all, you can finally say you know *Everything*®!

QUESTION

Answers to common questions

FACT

Important snippets of information

ALERT

Urgent warnings

ESSENTIAL

Quick handy tips

PUBLISHER Karen Cooper

DIRECTOR OF ACQUISITIONS AND INNOVATION Paula Munier

MANAGING EDITOR, EVERYTHING® SERIES Lisa Laing

COPY CHIEF Casey Ebert

ACQUISITIONS EDITOR Katrina Schroeder

SENIOR DEVELOPMENT EDITOR Brett Palana-Shanahan

EDITORIAL ASSISTANT Ross Weisman

EVERYTHING® SERIES COVER DESIGNER Erin Alexander

LAYOUT DESIGNERS Colleen Cunningham, Elisabeth Lariviere, Ashley Vierra, Denise Wallace

Visit the entire Everything® series at *www.everything.com*

THE EVERYTHING®
POST WEIGHT LOSS SURGERY COOKBOOK

All you need to meet and maintain
your weight loss goals

Jennifer Whitlock Heisler, RN

Foreword by Christine Ren Fielding, MD

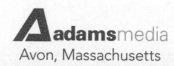
adamsmedia
Avon, Massachusetts

*Thank you to my wonderful husband Jeff. I couldn't have written
this book without your love, support, and culinary expertise.*

An Everything® Series Book.
Everything® and everything.com® are registered trademarks of F+W Media, Inc.

Published by Adams Media, a division of F+W Media, Inc.
57 Littlefield Street, Avon, MA 02322 U.S.A.
www.adamsmedia.com

ISBN 10: 1-4405-0386-9
ISBN 13: 978-1-4405-0386-3
eISBN 10: 1-4405-0387-7
eISBN 13: 978-1-4405-0387-0

Printed in the United States of America.

10 9 8 7 6 5 4 3 2

Library of Congress Cataloging-in-Publication Data
is available from the publisher.

This publication is designed to provide accurate and authoritative information with regard to the subject matter covered. It is sold with the understanding that the publisher is not engaged in rendering legal, accounting, or other professional advice. If legal advice or other expert assistance is required, the services of a competent professional person should be sought.

—From a *Declaration of Principles* jointly adopted by a Committee of the American Bar Association and a Committee of Publishers and Associations

Many of the designations used by manufacturers and sellers to distinguish their products are claimed as trademarks. Where those designations appear in this book and Adams Media was aware of a trademark claim, the designations have been printed with initial capital letters.

The information contained in this book is intended to communicate information which is helpful and educational to the reader. It is not intended to replace medical diagnosis or treatment, but rather to provide information and recipes which may be helpful in implementing a diet and program prescribed by your doctor. Please consult your physician for medical advice before changing your diet.

*This book is available at quantity discounts for bulk purchases.
For information, please call 1-800-289-0963.*

Contents

Acknowledgments

Thank you to my husband, Jeff, who helped with every aspect of the recipes provided in this book. Thank you to my Mom, Marti Miller, who told me over and over that I could accomplish anything I decided to do.

The Top 10 Things You Should Know about Weight Loss Surgery

1. Weight loss isn't easy, with or without surgery.

2. Losing weight can significantly boost your fertility.

3. Weight loss can reverse or improve type 2 diabetes, sleep apnea, high blood pressure, and high cholesterol.

4. Losing weight may improve your sex life.

5. Surgery is not without risks, but the health rewards may be well worth the possible complications.

6. You will be eating a low-fat, high-fiber, and high-protein diet, but that doesn't mean that your food can't be flavorful and appealing.

7. Weight loss can greatly reduce chronic pain.

8. You will need to exercise after surgery; eating right is not enough.

9. You may need to find a support group or seek out therapy to help you cope with all the changes caused by weight loss.

10. Cooking for yourself will help you control how many calories you are eating each day and can help you reach your goal weight.

Foreword

THE DECISION TO UNDERGO weight loss (or bariatric) surgery is a significant one. It requires courage to overcome feelings of failure and inadequacy, both self-perceived and reinforced by others. The biggest misconception is that obesity is a personal failing. This is founded on ignorance, and more importantly, poor understanding of the disease of obesity. Growing evidence shows that the wondrous nature of the human body changes its efficiency and energy storage mechanisms in relation to energy input. In other words, the body learns and accommodates to its intake of large portions of high calorie processed foods, and makes it practically impossible to accept a lower calorie intake. It's as hard as holding your breath for an hour. Your body gets starved for oxygen or gets starved for food.

While you are considering weight loss surgery, it is different than most other operations, because your disease does not end at the surgery. It is only the beginning. Surgery is only 50 percent of your success. What you do afterward is the other 50 percent of your success. Therefore you need to know what you are getting yourself into and how to make the best of your new tool.

This book is an excellent practical guide for anyone considering surgery, who has had surgery, or who loves them and wants to support them. This book provides much information to consider in your decision to have surgery; however, more importantly, you should use it as a guide for what to discuss with your surgeon during your decision-making process. Not all the information here is definitive because many surgeons do things a little bit differently. For example, the diet after surgery may be different; some ask you to stay on liquids for a week, some ask for a month. The hospital stay for each operation may vary according to your health condition, the type of operation, and your insurance policy.

If you have already had bariatric surgery, then this book will help you address many issues that may have developed or some that you may not even know are a problem! Perhaps you are confused as to why your husband keeps bringing home ice cream, why your mother keeps nagging you that you are getting too thin, or why you feel just plain angry. Much of the "untold stuff" that happens to many people after surgery is uncovered and can help you feel less weird about what you are feeling.

And finally, surgery is one of the best things you can do for yourself: health-wise, self-esteem–wise, job-wise, comfort-wise, social-wise and happiness-wise. After all your years of fighting to lose weight the "old-fashioned" way, surgery allows healthy eating, increased activity and exercise, and lifestyle changes to finally work! But it is not magic and the transition is not always easy. This book will give you tips on how to maximize your weight loss as well as your overall happiness.

—Christine Ren Fielding, MD
Director, NYU Program for Surgical Weight Loss

Introduction

WEIGHT LOSS SURGERY IS a very unique surgical procedure. With most surgeries, there is a problem, it is corrected by surgery, and once the recovery period ends, the problem is either fixed or improved. This cannot be said of weight loss surgery, because once the surgery is over, the real work begins, both physically and emotionally.

There is more to losing weight than finding a surgeon, being approved for surgery, and, finally, having the procedure. You will need to develop new coping skills, learn an entirely new way of eating, and make exercise a regular part of your life. For many, developing positive habits and breaking away from destructive old habits can be very challenging. You will need to cope with stress and daily struggles without reaching for food, but making these changes does get easier over time.

If you've never exercised before, you may be pleasantly surprised to find that you enjoy the activity and the stress relief that comes along with it. Taking an hour a day out of your busy life to exercise may provide multiple benefits. If you've been trying to find a way to make some "me time" in your life, this may be just what you have been looking for.

It isn't enough to limit the number of calories you take in on a daily basis. Many aspects of your life will need to change: the way you think about food, the way you cook, even the way you dress will change during the weight loss process.

Finding support, from friends, family, and even fellow weight loss surgery patients will be instrumental in your success. Finding someone who is willing to listen or someone who understands what you are going through is an invaluable part of the process. Your support system will help you get through the challenges you face, help you cope when you can no longer turn to food for comfort, and help you as you face an amazing number of changes.

It is safe to say that your life will be dramatically different after your surgery, mostly in very positive ways. As your body shrinks, you will find that you feel better, look better, have more energy, and can be a much healthier person than you ever imagined. If you have any doubt about how much better you will feel after your weight loss, pick up a sack of potatoes at the grocery store the next time you are shopping and see how long it takes before your arms get tired. You will be losing many times that weight, and no longer carrying those extra pounds with every step will feel fantastic.

None of these changes will happen without a great deal of hard work, but the rewards are well worth the effort. Fitting into smaller sizes, improving your self-confidence, and being able to go up a flight of stairs or out for a walk without being exhausted will be just a few of the rewards of your weight loss. While weight loss surgery isn't going to make all of your troubles go away, it may make health problems such as high blood pressure, sleep apnea, and type 2 diabetes disappear.

Things that you may have avoided in the past will become far easier as you lose weight. Imagine going to a movie and fitting comfortably into the movie seat, or taking a vacation to a sunny beach and wearing a bathing suit without feeling self-conscious. As you work toward your weight loss goal, you will be meeting other goals as well, such as being able to run and play with your children, or being able to walk from one end of the mall to the other without a second thought.

Plan on working hard to make your weight loss goals a reality, but know that your hard work will be rewarded in many ways, some expected, but many more that are unexpected and pleasant surprises.

CHAPTER 1

Introduction to
Weight Loss Surgery

If you are buying this book, you have made the decision to take some dramatic steps to improve your health and well-being. It can be a very scary decision, having surgery to lose weight, but it can also mean some very dramatic improvements in your life and how you feel. Surgery isn't for everyone, and there isn't even one particular weight loss procedure that is appropriate for everyone, but no one will argue that many people have amazing results after going forward with surgery.

Understanding Is Key

Becoming as knowledgeable as possible about your procedure, about the habits of successful weight loss surgery patients, and about yourself is tremendously important if you want to have a great outcome. The more you learn about what you can expect as a weight loss surgery patient, the more successful you will be.

It isn't enough to know what will be done during bariatric surgery, commonly known as weight loss surgery (WLS). Understanding the procedure you selected is important, and you should be thoroughly familiar with it; however, you will also need to think about your ideal diet after surgery, how to cook that diet or at least how to find appropriate items in a restaurant, and how to cope with the emotional issues that come with weight loss.

WLS is a process, and you will learn a great deal about yourself and your body as you work toward your weight loss goals. Don't discount the emotional part of weight loss, as identifying the reasons why you became overweight and learning how to cope with those emotions are keys to successfully losing weight and maintaining the loss.

You Are Not Alone

If you feel like you are the only person with a weight problem, think again. Obesity is a common issue, so much so that it has been labeled an epidemic by the World Health Organization. In the United States, almost one in three adults is obese, and the statistics are not improving. While obesity used to be a problem primarily faced by adults, now children are far more likely to be obese and are starting to face health issues that once only plagued older adults, such as high blood pressure, type 2 diabetes, and high cholesterol.

With the staggering numbers of overweight adults in America, it should be no surprise that record numbers of adults are seeking treatment. Reports indicate that $40 billion is spent annually on diets. That number includes formal programs for weight loss such as Weight Watchers and Jenny Craig, weight loss supplements, diet powders and shakes, and diet books, but does not include weight loss surgeries.

If those diet plans worked long term, the amount of money spent on weight loss could be justified. That just isn't the case. According to the *New England*

Journal of Medicine, most people regain a third of the weight they have lost dieting within a year, and are back at their original weight within three to five years. Most weight loss surgery patients have tried multiple diets, only to fail or to see the weight come back, sometimes even more weight than before.

ESSENTIAL

Recent studies show that 95 percent of dieters return to their starting weight within one to five years. Compare that with Roux-En-Y patients, who, on average, maintain a loss of 60–70 percent of their excess weight for ten years or longer.

By the time most people turn to weight loss surgery they have experienced years of frustration with diets and the inability to achieve lasting results.

Weight Loss Surgeries This Year

Almost 200,000 people will have a weight loss procedure this year, more than ever before, and that number promises to continue to increase as the benefits and long-term results associated with weight loss surgery are studied by the medical community and insurance companies. Men, women, and even teenagers are having surgery, and over 80 percent are doing so with coverage by their insurance company.

FACT

Adult women make up over 75 percent of weight loss surgery patients, but children (patients under the age of eighteen) and men are beginning to become a greater part of the bariatric surgery population.

In 2003 over 103,000 weight loss surgeries were performed, a number that has almost doubled in the years following. Why is surgery taking off as a method of weight control? Because studies and patients both are finding that surgery can work, not just for a month or a year, but for decades, for a lifetime. The Centers for Disease Control estimate that close to half a million people in America die each year due to obesity. This year, almost 200,000 people will decide that they don't want to die too young and that they want to live a healthy life, and weight loss surgery will help them do that.

If It Were Easy, Everyone Would Be Thin

Weight loss should be easy: Just burn more calories than you take in, right? Well, that is only one-tenth of the story. Weight loss is so much more complicated than a simple mathematical formula, and losing weight is never easy, surgery or not. While surgery is a powerful tool in the battle to lose weight, it still requires modification of the diet; exercise; and perhaps most importantly, some serious work on your personal relationship with food.

Contrary to what many think, weight loss surgery isn't the easy way out; it is merely the first step in the process. It isn't a decision that is made lightly, it requires a great deal of research and thought. It certainly isn't easy to qualify for a procedure, as some insurance companies resist paying for the expense of what is often considered an elective surgery.

ESSENTIAL

Current research shows that insurance companies recoup their investment in a patient's surgery within three to five years, as the patients become healthier and utilize their insurance less. The fact that weight loss surgery patients do keep the majority of their weight off in most cases, and in the end are less expensive to insure, should make the approval process easier in the future.

Losing Weight Is Hard Work

Weight loss can be a difficult process, and no matter how you do it the pounds don't fall off as if by magic. Losing weight, changing habits, exercising—none of these things are easy to do, and maintaining those changes is even more difficult. Getting up in the morning to get a workout in before work is not easy by any measure, but here's the bright side: It will get easier and become a habit. You will feel better as your body slims down and becomes stronger, giving you the motivation you need to keep getting on the treadmill.

Does surgery make it easier to lose weight? Certainly. But anyone who says that it is simple hasn't been through it. They haven't been through the early days of the liquid-only diet; they haven't been through the real work of figuring out why a stressful day at work leads to eating a full bag of potato chips; and they certainly don't understand what it is like to give up a favorite food because it ravages your system and makes you feel awful.

The Simple Truth about Weight Loss Surgery

Surgery is an amazing ally in the fight for good health, but the truth is that having surgery is a giant leap of faith. You are counting on results being worth any complications that you may have, that you will be able to overcome one bad day of overeating and get back on your program, and that your life will be made better. Many people will essentially mourn the loss of food, wishing for the comfort they feel when they eat certain things, but the results make it worthwhile to stay with the weight loss regime.

Life after Weight Loss Surgery

Life does change after weight loss surgery, usually for the better. Surgery won't make you rich, it won't improve a bad marriage, and it certainly won't improve how you sound when you sing in the shower, but it can make you healthier, much healthier.

It's easy to fall into the trap that everything will be wonderful after surgery. While it is fair to say that you will see a dramatic improvement in your life, you will still have problems, just like the people you know who are thin.

Weight Loss Surgery Myths

Misconceptions about weight loss surgery are so common that some weight loss surgery patients even believe them. It is important to get these myths out of the way, so the facts about weight loss procedures can be discussed.

EACH OF THESE STATEMENTS IS *FALSE*:

- Surgery is the easy way out.
- You will feel full after a few nibbles of food.
- You can't gain weight after weight loss surgery.
- Weight loss surgery is simple; there's no need to worry about complications.
- Your health conditions will disappear after surgery.
- Your body will be stunning after the weight is gone.
- Once you have lost the weight, your poor health conditions will never return.
- Your goal weight will be easy to attain.
- Your goal weight will be easy to maintain.
- Once you lose weight, all of your problems will be solved.
- Having the surgery will improve your marriage or relationship.
- You just eat less of the same things.
- Emotional eating stops after surgery.
- You don't need to exercise to lose weight.
- Surgery means never dieting again.
- You can't lose too much weight.
- Weight loss surgery is incredibly risky.
- Once you lose the weight, you can stop seeing your surgeon.

That's quite a list, isn't it? There are more myths out there, but these are among the most common. Did you see any that you thought were true? If you did, it is completely understandable. There is a great deal of misinformation about bariatric procedures out there. When in doubt, ask your surgeon.

Positive Changes in Store

If you've done research about what you can expect after surgery, you probably have heard the laundry list of good things that you can expect once you start losing weight, eating healthfully, and getting regular exercise. The news really is that good. Making the transition from obesity and a sedentary lifestyle to a more active and athletic lifestyle will mean much more than fitting into a smaller size.

The vast majority of bariatric patients have a comorbidity in addition to obesity, meaning that they have an additional health problem that can shorten their lifespan. The most common comorbidities are diabetes, sleep apnea, high cholesterol, and hypertension. Some patients have multiple comorbidities, making losing weight especially important. There is a light at the end of the tunnel. Study after study shows that patients who adhere to their doctor's instructions regarding diet and exercise see all of these conditions improve, and in many cases, resolve entirely. No more sleep apnea, no need for diabetes medications, cholesterol levels under control, blood pressure under control without medications—it isn't too good to be true. It is your reward for working hard to get healthy. The money you will save on prescriptions and visits to the doctor is just a bonus.

Pain? What Pain?

If you experience pain on a daily basis, you are not alone. Among the obese, chronic pain is common, the rule more than the exception. Joint pain, foot pain, and back pain can all be caused by carrying too much weight, and most pain resolves with weight loss. However, if you've had a back injury, weight loss may not make the pain go away entirely, but it certainly can't hurt! Weight loss surgery isn't a pain control surgery, but it is safe to say that if your weight is making your pain worse, then surgery has a great chance of improving your level of daily pain.

Breathe Better after Weight Loss

Breathing conditions are common among overweight individuals. Sometimes it is something as simple as being winded after climbing a flight of stairs, but others deal with asthma, sleep apnea, and other breathing issues. Some patients even require supplemental oxygen to make it through the day.

When you start losing weight, you may start to see your breathing condition improve dramatically. In fact, weight loss is so important to controlling sleep apnea that you may have to have your CPAP machine settings changed regularly, every time you lose ten to twenty pounds, because your breathing will improve as your body shrinks. Once you are well into your workout plan, you may be able to run up a flight of stairs without being short of breath, a very welcome change!

Shop Anywhere!

It may not be as important as being able to breathe easily or being able to stop taking medication every morning, but being able to shop in any store you like for clothing is a real benefit of weight loss. No more going to stores that only carry the largest of sizes; soon you will be able to shop in any clothing store.

ESSENTIAL

If you are having trouble resisting a tempting treat, close your eyes and imagine yourself buying a piece of clothing in a store that doesn't sell larger sizes. Imagine how it will feel to buy something in a much smaller size, and how good it will feel to wear that size.

Just imagine it—you are shopping for clothes in your regular "big" store and you realize that you can't fit into anything they are selling, because you are *too small!* It sounds like a dream doesn't it? It isn't a dream at all; many patients find that they no longer need plus-size or extra-large clothing after surgery, and they end up shopping in stores that they have never been able to shop in before.

Before Surgery

You haven't had surgery yet, but you are learning everything you can about what you should expect. Fantastic! Forewarned is forearmed. You will be glad you did a little extra homework to prepare for the big day. Surgery is hard enough without going into it unprepared.

If you've had surgery before, you may have a pretty realistic idea of what you should expect physically during your recovery, but a typical surgery doesn't present the emotional issues that weight loss surgery does. After your recovery is over, with a more typical surgery, you are back to your normal routine and activity, which is not the case with bariatric procedures. After the recovery is over, some of the hardest work begins.

Take the time to explore ways to make the process easier, clearing obstacles from your path before you meet them. Preparing for surgery and knowing exactly what to expect during a standard recovery may make it easier the first time your stomach is growling and you are only allowed to have a tablespoon of broth or a nibble of mashed potatoes because you are still recovering from your procedure. Doing your homework will also make it easier for you to start identifying the difference between "head hunger" and "stomach hunger" now, rather than after your procedure.

Start Exercising

Getting started on an exercise regime now will help you better tolerate your surgery and will help you get moving more quickly during your recovery. You don't have to be out running marathons to reap the rewards of exercise. Even a walk around the block is better than no exercise at all. If you don't exercise at all, try working up to half an hour of walking five days a week. Not only will you feel more energetic, but it will be easier to restart an existing exercise schedule after your procedure, rather than starting fresh.

ALERT

Is exercise painful because of your weight? Consider low- or no-impact exercise such as water aerobics or riding a bicycle. If you have trouble standing for periods of time, try doing the upper-body portion of a workout video while sitting. Every little bit of exercise helps!

Stop Smoking

If you are a smoker, you've probably heard it all before. Stop smoking to prevent cancer, wrinkles, and to reduce your risk of heart attack or stroke. What you may not know is that in addition to all the normal reasons for giving up cigarettes, stopping smoking four weeks before your procedure will reduce your risk of some very serious complications, including blood clots, having difficulty being weaned off of the ventilator, and poor wound healing. As a bonus, stopping smoking before your procedure can reduce the appearance of scars at your incision sites.

Line Up Your Support Team

If you are having surgery, you are going to need someone to drive you to and from the hospital. If you have children or pets, you will need some help there too, as you won't be able to lift anything heavier than five to ten pounds immediately after your surgery, and having a pet pulling you down the street on a walk could be downright painful.

If you have a spouse, friends, or family members who may be available to do some of the normal household work, it's time to ask them nicely if they would be willing to help out. You can expect to be tired after surgery, so arranging for child care and perhaps some light cooking during the first few days of your recovery at home is a great idea.

Get Groceries, Get Cooking

After surgery you're going to have some pain, and you can expect to be much more tired than usual. Why not prepare for your new diet by doing some grocery shopping before your surgery? You won't be able to lift bags of groceries right away, so shopping in advance can be truly helpful.

Once you have some groceries, you can prepare some food so that it is ready and waiting for you when you get home. Your diet will be limited initially, so whipping up some smoothies or some simple broths or soups before surgery will make your life easier later.

Fill Your Prescriptions

If your surgeon is willing to write the prescriptions that you will need after surgery before the procedure, take advantage of this opportunity to get them filled. You may not be able to drive in the days following your surgery, so having everything you need at home waiting for you will save you from finding someone to go to the pharmacy for you.

Identify Addictions

In addition to smoking, it is important that you address any other addictive behaviors that you may have. If you are actively using alcohol on a daily basis, or abusing drugs, these issues will not go away after surgery. If you are dependent upon drugs or alcohol, seek treatment before having surgery, as giving up an addiction to food can make other addictions significantly worse.

If you are experiencing addiction issues with food, it is also advisable to seek help before surgery. Take advantage of any therapy or support groups that your surgeon offers; your situation will be familiar to health care workers who work with bariatric patients on a regular basis.

ALERT

If you are using drugs and alcohol on a regular basis, going "cold turkey" during surgery and recovery can cause life-threatening problems such as seizures and withdrawal symptoms. Be sure to tell your surgeon if you regularly use drugs or alcohol.

Start a Food Diary

Before you have surgery, start writing down what you eat and drink and how much. Along with that vital information, jot down notes about how you were feeling when you ate. Were you hungry or just bored? Do you tend to overeat when you've had a stressful day at work? Are you more likely to eat healthfully if you work out in the morning? Do you eat badly when you're too tired to cook something that is healthy and nutritious?

Starting a food diary now may help you find patterns to your eating habits and identify the things that trigger overeating. The stressors that make you feel the urge to overeat will be present in your life after your surgery, so identifying them now will help you better cope when you are done with surgery and trying to create new and improved habits.

Get to Know Yourself Better

There are many questions you should be asking yourself in the quest to be well-prepared for the major life changes that happen after surgery. Can I handle going to a birthday party and skipping birthday cake, or should I consider not going and avoiding temptation? How should I reward myself for accomplishments if I can't do it with food? How will I celebrate my first ten-pound weight loss? Will my spouse or partner be supportive during this process?

Think about your life, the things you need to accomplish each day in addition to meeting your weight loss goals. Can you identify obstacles that are in your way? Are there things you can do today that will make it easier to start fresh with a healthy lifestyle, such as purchasing a gym membership?

Try to identify solutions to the problems you are aware of now, so that they aren't an issue once you are on the path to weight loss.

Get to Know Your Surgeon

If you are serious about having a weight loss surgery, then it is imperative that you also get serious about finding the right surgeon. Look for a surgeon who has not only performed hundreds, if not thousands of the bariatric procedures, but is also board certified in general surgery. Most bariatric surgeons are also members of the American Society of Bariatric Physicians or another group recognizing surgeons competent in bariatric medicine.

Don't hesitate to ask the surgeon questions about their training and qualifications to perform this type of surgery. If you have friends or acquaintances who have had weight loss surgery they can also be an excellent resource for finding a surgeon who will meet your expectations.

FACT

There are many bariatric surgery support forums available online. These can be a great place to learn more about your surgeon and how his patients feel about his bedside manner, skill, and the facility he uses for surgery.

Get to Know Your Surgery

Don't even consider having weight loss surgery if you don't understand the procedure. There are a wide variety of bariatric surgeries currently being performed, and you should be very knowledgeable about the procedure you have selected. In addition, you need to know the risks of the surgery, the potential complications (common and rare), and long-term results the average patient achieves with the procedure.

Eat Enough Protein

Protein is incredibly important before and after surgery. It is one of the most important nutrients when your body is working to heal your incisions and surgery sites. If you are deficient in protein, healing can be delayed and you may feel much more fatigued than you need to. After your surgery your body will have a greater need for protein than normal, so boosting your intake before surgery can help fill that need when you can't eat as much as your body requires.

Plan on eating a diet that is no less than 40 percent protein in the weeks leading up to surgery unless your surgeon has a specific plan for you to follow prior to surgery. Try to focus on lean protein such as chicken, low-fat dairy, and beans.

Give Up Caffeine

It's a lot to ask, but giving up caffeine prior to surgery will mean that you don't have terrible caffeine headaches during your recovery when your system won't tolerate coffee, tea, or soda. Try decreasing your intake slowly each day until you can go without caffeine completely the week before your surgery.

Recovering from surgery is hard enough without adding the symptoms of caffeine withdrawal, which include irritability, mild depression and anxiety, difficulty sleeping, headaches, fatigue, and difficulty concentrating. By cutting down slowly over a few weeks, the vast majority of caffeine withdrawal symptoms can be avoided entirely.

Plan for Time Away from Work

If you are currently working, don't forget to arrange for time away from work, whether you are taking vacation time, sick time, or just taking time away. You may need to produce paperwork from your surgeon in order to qualify for pay during your time away, so make sure you've completed the necessary paperwork well in advance of your surgery.

ALERT

If your job is physically strenuous or requires lifting, you may want to inform your surgeon. The typical estimates of time away from work may not be appropriate for someone who is very active in the workplace.

Obtain Birth Control

Plan on taking measures to prevent pregnancy if you are female, sexually active, and have not reached menopause. The weight loss that follows surgery can increase fertility in women significantly, but the first two years after the procedure are *not* the ideal time to become pregnant.

Talk to Someone Who Has Been There

If you do not know anyone who has been through bariatric surgery, your surgeon may be able to introduce you to patients who have had the procedure you have selected so that you may ask them about their experience. What do they wish they had known before surgery? What were they the most surprised by? Would they do it again? How did they like their surgeon? What would they change, if anything? What is the hardest part about life after weight loss surgery?

Don't be afraid to ask questions; most weight loss patients are very open about their surgeries as well as their experience after surgery, and most are more than willing to help other people who are considering doing the same thing.

Take Preoperative Instructions Seriously

When you are given your preoperative instructions, they are meant to be followed to the letter, including when you can and cannot eat or drink. You may have to do "bowel prep" prior to your surgery, which typically involves drinking a special fluid that will remove all food and stool from your system. Most patients experience liquid stool or diarrhea during the prep process. After completing prep, you will not be able to eat without increasing your risk of infection and other complications.

FACT

Eating or drinking before your surgery increases your risk of aspirating, or breathing fluid into your lungs, which can cause pneumonia. Avoid breathing problems after surgery by following your surgeon's instructions and not eating food or drinking fluids before your procedure.

Some people feel lightheaded or experience stomach cramping or nausea when taking the bowel prep medications. If you do, you might need to drink the medication more slowly in order to prevent your symptoms from worsening.

You may be told to stop drinking at a certain time the evening before surgery. The only exception to that will be taking medications with small sips of water the morning of surgery.

Which Meds Should I Take?

During your last preoperative visit with your surgeon, plan on discussing which medications you should or should not take prior to surgery if you are currently taking prescription medications. If you routinely take over-the-counter medications, those should be discussed with the surgeon as well. Some medications, such as insulin or other diabetic drugs, can cause problems if they are taken without food.

If your medications are taken in pill form, plan to take them with the least amount of water possible, as eating and drinking before surgery can create a risk of choking or aspirating food and fluid during the procedure. Vitamins and other over-the-counter supplements should not be taken before surgery unless expressly permitted by the surgeon and the anesthesia provider who will be present during surgery.

Paying Cash for Surgery

If your insurance company is not helping pay for your surgery and you are making arrangements to pay for surgery yourself, make sure that aftercare is included in the contract. Your surgeon may quote you a price for surgery that "includes everything," but that may not include both emotional support and the medical support you need after your procedure. Make sure that office visits after your surgery are included in the fee, as well as any scheduled counseling, therapy, or support groups that are given to patients with surgery paid for by insurance.

CHAPTER 2

Recovering from Your Surgery

Weight loss procedures are unique for one huge reason: Patients are actually happy and excited to have the surgery. That doesn't change the fact that there is still a recovery period, with the discomfort, challenges, and potential complications that all surgery patients face, along with issues that are unique to weight loss procedures.

A Typical Recovery

A normal recovery from weight loss surgery typically lasts four to six weeks. That is the time it takes your body to fully heal your incisions, internally and externally, and bounce back from the physical stress of the procedure. While the tissue that was operated upon won't be full strength for up to six months, most surgery patients are able to resume their normal activity, including working, exercising, having sex, and lifting heavy objects within two months, often much sooner with some of the less invasive procedures.

During your recovery, your body will be undergoing a remarkable transformation. In addition to healing your skin and muscle where the incisions were made, your body will be growing accustomed to a very different lifestyle, as your eating and exercise habits change dramatically. It is normal to feel somewhat uncomfortable with your own body in the first few weeks or months after surgery. So much is changing, from what you can eat to when you can drink, and it will take time to adapt to your new lifestyle changes.

Waking Up in the Hospital

Your surgery is over, it's time to get on with your weight loss plans, right? Well, yes and no. It's time to recover from your surgery and get back on your feet so you can feel 100 percent and truly get started with your weight loss plans.

Once your surgery is over, you will wake up in one of two places; in a special unit in the hospital called the Post-Anesthesia Care Unit (PACU), otherwise known as the recovery room, or you may be in your assigned hospital room. If you wake up in the PACU, once you're completely awake and your condition is stable, you will be taken to your hospital room.

The vast majority of weight loss surgeries require at least one night in the hospital. For some of the more complex procedures several days may be appropriate. During this time, your surgeon and the nursing staff will be observing your condition closely, looking for any signs or symptoms of complications. You may be monitored with a pulse oximeter, a device that measures the amount of oxygen in your bloodstream, or even a heart monitor, which will display your heart rhythms.

Your body will still be working to clear the anesthesia medications during your first day after surgery, so feeling groggy or sleeping most of the day is normal. Don't be surprised if you are awakened periodically to have your temperature taken or to check your vital signs. The staff may even wake you to see if you need pain medication so that your medication doesn't completely wear off while you sleep, causing you to wake up with significant pain.

ESSENTIAL

To help monitor your pain, hospital staff use a pain scale. The scale is from zero to ten, with zero being no pain and ten being the most excruciating pain you've ever experienced. Staff will ask about your level of pain before medication, then again after the medication takes effect, to help determine the most appropriate dose of the pain reliever.

The second day after surgery is typically the most painful. You will feel sore and you may require pain medication, even if you didn't the day of surgery. Your stomach and abdomen will be particularly sore, but your back may also be sore from lying flat on the operating table.

Get Up and Get Moving

Most surgeons expect their patients to be up and walking within eight to twelve hours of surgery. That doesn't mean that you will be marching up and down the hallways for hours immediately after your procedure, but a trip from your bed to the bathroom, or a few steps down the hallway, should be expected. Getting up and moving can help prevent serious complications, including blood clots and pneumonia, making it a very important part of the recovery process.

As excited as you must be to get started on your weight loss regime, it is important not to overdo your physical activity immediately after surgery. Walking is a great low-impact exercise that is completely appropriate during your recovery. Swimming is also low impact, but should wait until your incisions have completely closed. High-impact exercise and rigorous activity that could put stress on your healing incisions should wait for clearance from your physician.

How Much Exercise During Recovery?

Your best guide to what amount of exercise is appropriate for you is your level of pain and fatigue. Does walking cause minimal pain as long as you limit your walk to less than twenty minutes? Or does walking down the hall to the bathroom exhaust you and leave you breathless? If you are able to do a few minutes of walking, do a few minutes and then do more the next day. If there is no good reason not to walk around your neighborhood for half an hour, then get out there and do it!

Even if you are feeling great, if you are still in recovery and this is your first time attempting exercise, take it easy. What feels great during the workout may not feel so good the next day when muscle soreness sets in. Be moderate in your activity until you are sure that you won't suffer for it the next day.

Exercises to Avoid During Recovery

Weight training and lifting objects weighing more than five to ten pounds should not be done for the first two weeks after surgery. Do not attempt any strenuous exercise, full-impact exercise, or lifting until you have seen your surgeon and have been released to return to work and resume full physical activity.

Exercise is important, and getting started right away is the expectation for most patients, as long as the type of exercise is appropriate for someone recovering from surgery. It is absolutely true that the sooner you start exercising, the sooner you will start losing weight, but choosing a type of exercise that does not harm your healing body is essential.

Eating During Your Recovery

Your first "food" after surgery will be clear liquids, most likely water. Starting with small sips, you will see if you can tolerate small amounts without becoming nauseated or vomiting. Once you are able to tolerate clear liquids without difficulty, a full liquid diet will start, which includes broths and other flavored liquids. If a full liquid diet is tolerated, pureed foods such as smoothies are next, followed by soft foods, and finally a diet of regular foods.

This progression from liquids to small amounts of solid food may happen over the course of days, or even over many weeks, depending on the type of surgery. Gastric banding patients typically recover and eat a full diet much more quickly than bypass patients, who have had surgical changes made to their stomach and small intestine.

ALERT

After weight loss surgery you should limit your fluid intake at meal times. In addition to refraining from drinking during your meal, you should not have any fluids thirty minutes before or after a meal. Combining food and fluids can lead to discomfort, nausea, and vomiting, as well as feeling full from a meal because you've had too much to drink.

It is important to remember that all of these foods will be taken in far smaller quantities than you were accustomed to prior to your surgical procedure. Once you are able to tolerate more than fluid, start with a few nibbles of food, wait for a few minutes, then take a few more nibbles if you are still interested and feeling good. You will find that you feel satiated with far less food than you did prior to surgery, so it is very important to listen to your body and stop eating when you have a sensation of fullness.

FACT

If you've had gastric bypass surgery, your first meals after surgery will be very small. Your new stomach pouch will have a small capacity, possibly as little as thirty to sixty milliliters (two to four tablespoons) and won't tolerate being stretched with food or fluids early in the recovery period.

Foods to Avoid During Recovery

During your recovery you will want to stay away from any foods that might irritate your stomach, cause diarrhea, or discomfort. Even if you are able to tolerate regular foods, the texture of your food will be more important than ever before. Potato chips are a great example of a food to avoid after surgery. Not only are they full of fat and empty calories, but the texture is all wrong for someone recovering from surgery. The hard, sharp edges can cause significant pain when the chip reaches your stomach. The same is true of healthier foods that are also hard, such as carrots.

Foods that cause constipation, such as cheese, should also be avoided. Foods that upset your stomach prior to surgery or gave you gas could cause pain during your recovery. Your system is likely to be more sensitive to food choices after surgery than ever before, so avoid anything that has caused problems in the past.

Sugar and Dumping Syndrome

Sugar is an important food to avoid for weight loss surgery patients. Not only is it full of calories and lacking in nutrition, it can be very upsetting to the stomach. For gastric bypass patients, sugar is responsible for "Dumping Syndrome," or rapid gastric emptying. After eating foods with sugar, the food will pass out of the stomach and into the intestine much more rapidly than is normal, or "dump."

Dumping may be accompanied by lightheadedness, nausea, fatigue, sweating, diarrhea, and even heart palpitations. Hypoglycemia, or low blood sugar, often occurs along with other symptoms. Dumping syndrome typically starts forty-five minutes after a meal, and resolves within a few hours.

Foods to Eat During Recovery

Once you are able to tolerate your liquid diet without difficulty and are ready to move on to pureed or soft foods, stick with foods that are easily digested until you know how your body will handle the change. Smoothies and mashed potatoes (skin off) are a great way to see if you are able to tolerate the move from liquids to soft foods. Just because it has to be pureed or soft doesn't mean you have to eat baby food! There are many ways to include foods in your new diet that aren't unappetizingly bland. Your food can be full of flavor, even if it doesn't have to be chewed as much as a standard meal. See Chapter 14 for soft food recipes.

When Can You Go Home?

Your doctor will want to be sure that you are able to care for yourself and that your bodily functions have returned to normal before discharging you. The surgeon will want to be sure that you are not having any serious complications, and if you are having minor or treatable side effects from the surgery, that you have been given the tools you need to continue recovering successfully.

The doctor may want to run some blood tests, just to make sure there are no signs of bleeding, infection, or any other problems that should be treated while you are in the hospital. Blood tests are routinely done after surgery, so this should not be alarming.

Are You Ready to Go Home?

There are a few key factors that will determine if you are able to go home from the hospital, including:

- You are able to walk without assistance, if you were able to prior to surgery.
- You are able to urinate without difficulty.
- You have had a bowel movement or passed gas.
- You are able to tolerate fluids without vomiting.
- Your vital signs are normal, including your temperature.
- No signs of serious complications are present.
- You have a responsible adult available to drive you home.

Important Discharge Information

Being discharged from the hospital may feel like cause for celebration. It is a rare person who would rather be in the hospital than in their own home. Before you dash out the door, it is important that you make sure you have everything you need to have a successful recovery. If you have questions that have not been answered, this is the time to speak up. The surgeon and the nurses are your best resources for information about what you should be doing, what you can expect, and how to make the most of your weight loss goals.

What You Need Before You Go Home

When you do receive the news that you are going home, there are four things that you will need to take home with you:

- **Discharge instructions.** These are the doctor's rules regarding what you can eat, how much you can eat and any other rules or expectations he has for you until your first follow-up visit. A staff member should discuss these instructions with you in detail, answering any questions you may have.
- **Prescriptions.** If you were unable to fill your prescriptions prior to your surgery, they should be given to you at the time of discharge or phoned in to your pharmacy.
- **Follow-up care arrangements.** Your first appointment with your doctor should be scheduled at this time or instructions for making the appointment should be provided.
- **Emergency contact information.** When you leave the hospital, you should be provided with at least one way to contact your surgeon, or the surgeon's staff, in case of an emergency.

Once you have answers to your important surgery questions, and you've been given the information you need, you're ready to continue recovering in the comfort of your own home!

Incision Care after Surgery

Proper care of your incisions is very important to prevent infection and minimize scarring. Most patients have laparoscopic incisions—several small incisions approximately half an inch in length—which are common with minimally invasive procedures. A small minority of patients have "open" procedures, with full-length incisions.

Small incisions are often closed with surgical glue or small adhesive bandages, rather than sutures. In some cases, if the incision is in an area where there might be a great deal of movement of the skin, or the incision may have tension placed upon it, a small number of staples or sutures may be placed to provide extra support. Larger incisions are typically closed with staples, then covered with a sterile bandage.

While you are in the hospital, the nursing staff will help care for your incisions. You may not want to look at your incisions, but watching as nurses provide wound care will help when you return home, because you can observe how they treat the incision and do the same. You will also know how your incisions looked in the hospital, so you aren't left wondering if they look the same as when the nurses said you were healing normally.

ALERT

One of the most important things you can do to protect your incision is to always wash your hands before touching it. This will help prevent your hands from contaminating your incision as long as you wash your hands thoroughly, scrubbing with soap for at least thirty seconds.

Inspecting Your Incision

Each day you will want to inspect your incisions. You will need to make sure each incision is clean and look for signs of infection, signs of healing, and any indications that the incision is pulling apart instead of healing. Your incision should show small signs of improvement each day or two, with the redness decreasing and the incision growing smaller as it heals.

In the first days of recovery a small amount of clear fluid may be present on the incision, and scabs are normal during the healing process, but there should be no bloody drainage or pus coming from the incision. If the incision appears to be pulling apart, or if there is abnormal drainage present, notify your surgeon.

Cleaning Your Incision

The easiest way to clean your incision each day is to do it in the shower. Using a gentle antibacterial soap, lather and rinse the area as you would any other area of your body. Do not scrub the area to remove scabs or the adhesive bandages; both should be allowed to fall off on their own. If the adhesive bandages are still in place fourteen days after surgery and your wound has completely closed, they can be peeled off gently while in the shower, or your physician can remove them at your follow-up appointment.

Resist the temptation to use harsh solutions such as peroxide and alcohol, which will dry out the incision and can lead to irritation. Lotions, ointments, and powders should also be avoided, including antibacterial ointments used for cuts and scrapes, unless your surgeon specifically instructs you otherwise.

If you have sutures or staples, you will want to make sure that they are still in place and holding the incision firmly closed. Do not attempt to clean the individual staples or sutures: Focus on keeping the wound itself clean rather than what is keeping the wound closed.

Scars and Incisions

If you are concerned about scars from your surgery there are several things that can help minimize the lasting effects on your skin. Preventing infection is one of the best ways to minimize the scars: An infection slows healing and can result in much more severe scarring than would be present otherwise. Refrain from picking at or scrubbing the incision and any scabs that may be present.

Minimizing exposure to the sun is also helpful in reducing how noticeable the incisions will be. Keep them covered or apply sunscreen once they are fully healed, to prevent sun damage to the area.

One of the best ways to prevent scarring is to stop smoking. Smoking slows healing significantly and has been shown to increase scarring. Stopping smoking at least two weeks prior to surgery will not only reduce your risk of scarring, it will also reduce your risk of serious complications such as blood clots and pneumonia.

There are over-the-counter medications available to reduce the appearance of scars, but they should not be used until the incision closes completely. If you have a history of scarring badly and are concerned about further scarring, discuss the situation with your physician. There are prescription medications and treatments available to minimize and prevent scars after surgery.

Signs of Emergency after Surgery

All surgeries have a risk of complications, and weight loss surgery is no exception. As many as one in ten weight loss surgery patients experience a minor or major complication, so it is important to know what symptoms indicate a normal recovery from surgery and which ones should be more alarming. For example, after surgery some pain is expected and should be considered perfectly normal; however, sudden, excruciating pain that cannot be controlled would not be considered normal.

Emergencies are rare after weight loss surgery; only 2–3 percent of patients ever experience a life-threatening complication, but early identification of a problem is essential. If you believe you are having a complication that is a potential emergency, do not hesitate to contact your surgeon. You may be tempted to wait until the next morning if it is late at night, but it is not advisable to do so.

If you do decide to go to the emergency room, you will need to explain very clearly that you have had a recent weight loss procedure. For example, "I had Roux-En-Y gastric bypass surgery two weeks ago, performed by Dr. Smith. I was discharged from Jones Hospital ten days ago. I am here because I was told that if I noticed any shortness of breath I should report to the emergency room and have the staff contact the doctor immediately." Knowing your recent surgical history will be helpful to the staff as they work to determine the nature of your problem.

Bleeding after Surgery

For gastric bypass procedures a small amount of blood in the stool in the first few days after surgery is not unheard of, but you should make your surgeon aware of it, as it is not typical. Any other bleeding, such as vomiting blood or bleeding from incisions, should be reported to the surgeon immediately. Stool that is dark in color and tarry in appearance also indicates the presence of blood and should be reported.

Difficulty Breathing

Shortness of breath or difficulty breathing should never be ignored. Unexplained shortness of breath can indicate a major complication, such as a blood clot in the lungs, so reporting this symptom to your surgeon is absolutely essential. If the difficulty is severe, consider calling 911 and seeking treatment from emergency medical technicians (EMTs), rather than waiting to hear from your surgeon.

ALERT

If you are experiencing a surgical emergency, do not drive yourself to the emergency room. It is better to call an ambulance and have care from trained professionals on the way to the hospital than to take the risk of becoming more seriously ill during the drive.

Blood Clots

Deep vein thrombosis (DVT) is the name given to blood clots that occur after surgery. Blood clots typically form in the legs, but they can form in other locations, or they can move through the bloodstream to form a clot elsewhere. Leg pain, along with redness and warmth over the site of pain, cramping, and numbness can indicate that a blood clot has occurred. In some cases, the affected leg may be larger than the other, as blood begins to "back up" in the limb.

Patients who have experienced blood clots in the past are at greater risk for a clot than patients who have never had one. Clots are considered a medical emergency because they can cause tissue damage in the affected limb, but they can also travel to the vessels of the lungs, causing a pulmonary embolus, or to the brain, causing a stroke.

Suture Line Disruption (SLD)

Suture line disruption is the medical term for a line of sutures or staples that is no longer intact, with one or more of the stitches or staples coming loose. It can occur in bypass procedures such Roux-En-Y, where the anatomy of the body has been changed, and in procedures that alter the size of the stomach. It does not occur in gastric banding patients.

SLD can allow food and fluids to move out of the GI tract, possibly causing a life-threatening infection to develop. This complication typically presents as a significant increase in pain and may be accompanied by a fever if an infection has started. Blood may also be present in the stool.

Complications and Side Effects after Surgery

Complications after surgery are not uncommon, but they can be annoying and may slow your recovery. Some issues may not be noticeable until after your recovery and just when you thought you were back to your old self and well on your way to significant weight loss.

Many of these problems can be prevented entirely with some planning, and the problems that can't be prevented may seem less alarming if you are aware in advance that they can happen.

Common Side Effects after General Anesthesia

Weight loss surgeries are performed under anesthesia, meaning that you are asleep for the entire procedure, and you are given medication that prevents your muscles from moving during the procedure. The muscles that help the lungs inhale and exhale are affected by general anesthesia, so a breathing tube and a ventilator are required to provide the patient with oxygen while the procedure is being done.

After general anesthesia the following are common:

- **Sore throat.** The insertion of the breathing tube, and having it in place for several hours, can be very irritating to the throat. Normal sore throat remedies, such as lozenges, are appropriate to relieve the irritation.
- **Difficulty urinating.** During surgery, a catheter is placed in the bladder to empty urine throughout the procedure. The insertion can be irritating to the urethra, the tube that takes urine from the bladder to the outside of the body. The bladder can also be slow to "wake up" from general anesthesia, making it difficult to urinate.
- **Constipation.** The medication used to paralyze your muscles during surgery also paralyzes the muscular walls of the intestine. If those

muscles are slow to wake, constipation can result. The use of prescription pain medications also contributes to constipation. Constipation should be treated immediately and may require over-the-counter or prescription medication, based on your surgeon's recommendation. Gastric bypass patients are especially sensitive to constipation, as it can cause stress on the areas where the rerouted intestines are placed.

Walking regularly and staying hydrated can help prevent constipation, along with eating a diet high in fiber when you are able.

FACT

In some rare cases, a segment of the intestine does not "wake up" from anesthesia as it should, a complication called an ileus. It is more common in surgeries that take place in the abdomen, and even more common in surgeries that require the intestines to be manipulated, such as gastric bypass. Medication can be given to treat the problem, but no eating or drinking is allowed until the problem resolves.

Pain after Surgery

Some pain is normal after surgery, but surgical pain tends to start improving on the second or third day after surgery, and slowly improve each day thereafter. Stomach pain after surgery can be caused by a variety of things. Sudden, excruciating pain should never be ignored, but less severe pain may have a variety of causes.

Some common causes of pain after weight loss surgery include:

- Carbonated drinks such as soda
- Progressing from a liquid diet to a normal diet too quickly
- Eating too much food at one time
- Eating too quickly
- Drinking through a straw
- Drinking too much fluid at one time

- Stomach gas, caused by gas-producing foods such as cucumbers or beans
- Drinking while eating
- Vomiting
- Reflux, also known as heartburn
- Eating food that is irritating to the stomach too soon
- Incision pain from not supporting the incision while coughing, standing up, or sneezing
- Difficulty swallowing, caused by overly large bites or not chewing well enough

FACT

A bland diet is necessary immediately after surgery. Many foods that you enjoyed prior to surgery can be very irritating to the stomach during the recovery phase. Foods that are most likely to cause stomach pain and irritation include acidic foods, such as tomatoes and lemons; hard or crunchy foods, such as carrots; spicy foods; and foods high in sugar.

The Stress of Surgery

Surgery is stressful, both physically and emotionally. All that stress can slow your healing in a number of ways, interfering with your ability to get a good night's rest, slowing wound healing, and making your recovery feel like an emotional roller coaster. Minimizing your stress level makes sense for both your mind and body. Just because you are recovering from surgery doesn't mean you can't do some of the things you normally would to relax. A good book, a spa day, or a movie with friends is just as relaxing after surgery as it was before surgery. Take the time to take care of yourself emotionally while you are recovering physically; it is well worth the effort.

Don't be shocked if you find yourself craving foods that you know you cannot have during your recovery. If you are someone who typically eats when you are stressed, it is especially important that you find new ways to cope, because eating the wrong foods during your recovery will not only sabotage your weight loss efforts, it could cause serious pain when your system can't handle the food.

CHAPTER 3

Types of Weight Loss Surgery and Special Needs

Not all weight loss surgeries are the same. The potential complications vary from procedure to procedure, just as the surgeon's instructions will vary widely. It is important to know what type of surgery you had, what complications you should be looking for, and how you can help prevent discomfort and problems.

Restrictive Procedures

Restrictive weight loss procedures are surgeries that promote weight loss by decreasing the amount of food that can be eaten. This is done in a variety of ways, including decreasing the size of the stomach, placing a band around the entrance to the stomach, and dividing the stomach into parts using staples to decrease the volume the stomach can hold.

These procedures are known by a variety of names. You may hear them referred to as "gastric banding," "sleeve procedures," "stomach stapling," "gastroplasty," or "bariatric surgery."

Gastric banding surgeries are the most popular type of restrictive procedures today, and are also known by a variety of names and brands, including Lap-Band and Realize band. This surgery places an adjustable band around the top of the stomach, which slows the ingestion of food and dramatically reduces the amount of food that can be taken in during a meal.

Additional types of restrictive surgeries include vertical banded gastroplasty; vertical gastric sleeve, which surgically creates a smaller stomach that is tube-shaped; and "stomach stapling" a procedure that is no longer performed on a regular basis.

Restrictive procedures are less invasive than malabsorptive procedures, as the surgery is performed only on or around the stomach, typically using laparoscopic, or minimally invasive, techniques. These procedures work by decreasing the size of the stomach, which creates a feeling of fullness with far less food.

Bypass Weight Loss Surgery

Malabsorptive weight loss surgeries are procedures that cause weight loss by decreasing the amount of calories the body is able to absorb. This is done by rerouting the gastrointestinal system to bypass a significant portion of the small intestine, the part of the body that absorbs nutrients from food.

In reality, the surgeries that are referred to as "malabsorptive" are actually a combination of restrictive surgeries that reduce the amount of food that can be eaten and the malabsorptive component, but for clarity, the surgeries are referred to as "malabsorptive surgeries." They are known by a wide variety of names including "bypass surgery," "Roux-En-Y," "Duodenal Switch," "Biliopancreatic Diversion," and the general term "bariatric surgery."

Malabsorptive procedures are more invasive than the restrictive surgeries, as they require additional procedures to be performed on the small intestine. The increased amount of incisions increases the risk of the procedure, but the end result may be worth it for many patients, as the overall weight loss tends to be greater for patients having bypass surgeries.

Special Considerations after Restrictive Surgery

After having restrictive weight loss surgery, there are some unique challenges that patients face. These side effects are typically more annoying than serious, but should be noted and avoided when possible. Restrictive surgery, unlike bypass surgery, does not alter the way the body absorbs calories, so malnutrition is typically not an issue.

Many people think that complications from surgery only happen to other people, but being aware of the potential for problems can help you spot an issue before it becomes a major health concern. If you are concerned about a symptom that you are experiencing, or if you think something just isn't right, speak to your physician.

Chew, Chew, and Chew Again

After having a restrictive surgery (and since bypass surgeries have a restrictive component, this pertains to all bariatric patients) it is imperative that you take the time to chew your food very thoroughly, not swallowing until your food is the consistency of paste. This will considerably slow the rate at which you eat, which is a good thing when trying to lose weight, but it will also make sure that you don't have the uncomfortable, and sometimes painful, experience of food lodging at the bottom of your esophagus.

ESSENTIAL

How much chewing is enough? Plan on chewing every nibble-sized bite twenty to thirty times, until the food is paste-like. This will prevent having food feel "stuck" or cause pain with sharp edges. Over time, chewing your food this way will become a habit and you won't have to think about it or count how many times you chew.

Early after your surgery your stomach may be sensitive to food, and chewing food very thoroughly will help ease you through your recovery. Hard or crunchy food can be especially irritating and sometimes painful, so chewing these foods well is doubly important.

Band Adjustments

If you have had a gastric banding surgery, your band will have to be adjusted periodically to achieve the best results, a procedure commonly referred to as a "fill." Your band is a hard outer shell with an internal bladder similar to an inner tube. In most cases, the inner tube is empty following surgery, allowing your stomach time to recover from surgery before restricting the passage of food.

Inflating the inner portion of the band increases the restriction you feel when you eat. Your first fill will be done at the discretion of your surgeon. Some prefer to wait until you are able to eat a normal diet for at least a week; others complete the first fill six to eight weeks after the surgery.

The procedure is a simple one, but will require some minor preparation on your part. Typically, no food should be eaten the day of surgery, so you will need to stop eating the evening before the procedure. Fluids are acceptable and help flush your stomach, so small quantities are encouraged before your fill takes place.

A gastric band has a port that allows it to be filled with sterile saline or to release saline to deflate the inner bladder. The port rests under your skin and in some individuals can be felt when pressing gently over the stomach. Accessing the port through the skin does require a needle, but is generally not a painful process.

Before your fill begins your skin will be cleaned using a special solution that reduces the chances of infection and may also be shaved in a small area over your stomach. Then, using fluoroscopy to visualize your band and the port on the band, a needle will be inserted into your skin and into the port on the band. Saline can be injected into the port, or removed via the port, depending on the needs of the patient.

The entire process typically takes fifteen minutes or less and can be repeated as necessary. Two or three fills are typically adequate for most patients to get the level of restriction they require to effectively lose weight.

After your fill it may take a few days to get used to the new adjustment, and you will have to take care not to overeat or swallow large pieces of food. After a fill, you should find that you feel full more quickly than you did immediately prior to the fill.

FACT

Fluoroscopy is similar to an X-ray, but shows structures of the body in real time, like a video. Using this technique, your surgeon can see the port of your gastric band and the needle he is using. Not only is the fill completed quickly, the surgeon is able to see if the band is as full as it should be, and make corrections immediately if necessary.

Focus on Changing Habits

To be successful after a restrictive surgery your habits must change. Unlike bypass surgery, restrictive surgeries don't change the amount of calories your body can utilize, it just encourages you to eat less. If you have surgery and you don't reduce your food intake you will not meet your weight loss goals.

Overeating can be painful with restrictive surgeries, and it can also cause pouch stretching, which means the tiny stomach the surgeon made will expand over time, accommodating larger and larger meals. In order to prevent pouch stretching, it is important to avoid drinking with meals, eating a larger quantity of food than your surgeon recommends, and most importantly, avoiding foods that provide calories with little nutritional value.

Feelings of Tightness

Gastric bands may feel tighter in the morning and much looser as the day progresses. You may also find that the band becomes tighter at certain times of the month, such as the week before your menstrual period. Generally speaking, if something makes your fingers swell and your rings feel tight, it may also make your gastric band feel tighter.

Restrictive Surgery as First Step

For some patients who are extremely obese—having a BMI of 60 or greater—a restrictive surgery may be the first step in treatment. These patients may be too heavy to tolerate the more invasive bypass procedures, or have other medical conditions that make the surgery inadvisable. In these cases it is better to have a restrictive surgery to help them reduce their body size so that they are able to have a bypass procedure later.

ESSENTIAL

Your BMI, or body mass index, is a measure of body fat. A BMI of 18.5 to 24.9 is considered normal, 25–29.9 is overweight, and greater than 30 is obese. A BMI of 30 or greater is required by most surgeons for a patient to be a candidate for surgery.

For patients who have bariatric surgery in two steps, the total weight loss goal may be much greater than what can be reasonably lost with restrictive procedures alone. To meet the final goal, bypass surgery will be required, and even then the long-term goal may be to reach a BMI that is still in the obese category.

Special Considerations after Bypass Surgery

Bypass surgery comes with all the potential complications that affect patients who have restrictive surgeries, along with some additional issues. Bypass surgeries are more complex than banding surgeries, and because of this, complications are more likely. The bypass procedure also alters the way food is digested, so some stomach upset may be present after surgery.

Dumping Syndrome

If you've had bypass surgery, you've probably heard a great deal about the potential for having dumping syndrome. Food or liquids, typically those heavy in sugar, cause food to rapidly move from your stomach and into your small intestine, or "dump." If you've had a procedure that removes the pylorus, or sphincter muscle at the bottom of the stomach, you will be more likely to experience dumping syndrome. Diabetics, patients who have had the vagus nerve to their stomach severed, and patients who have had surgery to reduce reflux (heartburn) are also at increased risk.

ALERT

Beware of hidden sugars in food. Many fat-free and low-fat foods replace fat with sugar to improve the flavor. Foods that don't taste sweet, such as tomato sauce, often contain much more sugar than you might expect. Plan on reading labels when you shop if you are prone to dumping syndrome.

Dumping syndrome is typically not harmful, but the symptoms can be alarming and painful. In rare cases, dumping can cause fainting, confusion, and heart palpitations.

COMMON SYMPTOMS OF DUMPING SYNDROME:

- Nausea and vomiting
- Weakness
- Stomach cramps
- Sweating
- Lightheadedness
- Bloating
- Belching
- Diarrhea
- Rapid heart rate
- Low blood glucose (blood sugar)

Dumping is often referred to as "early dumping" or "late dumping." Early pertains to dumping syndrome that happens immediately after a meal while late dumping happens an hour or longer after a meal.

Tiny Meals and Pouch Capacity

After a bypass procedure, the volume of food you are able to eat will be drastically reduced. A normal stomach can hold anywhere from one to two quarts of food and fluid comfortably, and can stretch to accommodate even more when necessary. After bypass surgery, your stomach capacity may be as little as thirty milliliters, or two tablespoons of food or liquid. More food than that can be very uncomfortable and can place stress upon the incisions made in your stomach.

In the days and weeks immediately after surgery, it can take a great deal of effort to drink the recommended sixty-four ounces of water per day. Fluid will have to be taken in sips, and food will have to be nibbled in small amounts and be well chewed.

Over time the capacity of your stomach will increase, but it is a slow process. Most patients are able to eat one cup of food at a time within three months of surgery after slowly increasing meal sizes each week. When meals are this small, it is very important to make every morsel count, choosing lean, high-protein foods and avoiding empty calories at all costs. It is important to remember that these small meals will be surprisingly satisfying, providing a feeling of fullness, due to the decrease in the size of your stomach's capacity.

Long-Term Issues after Restrictive Surgery

After you have fully healed from your surgery and are well on your way to reaching your weight loss goals, it may feel as though the potential for complications from your surgery has passed. While the majority of serious complications do occur during the recovery period, there are still complications that can happen in the months and years after surgery.

Gastric Erosion and Band Erosion

The terms "gastric erosion" and "band erosion" are often used interchangeably, but they are not the same condition. Gastric erosion is an ulcer, eroding an area of tissue of the stomach. This condition can occur in people who have not had weight loss surgery, but may be more common in those who do.

Patients who have gastric banding are at risk for having the band erode the muscular stomach wall, called band erosion. The band is a foreign body, and with each swallow and muscle contraction of the stomach, the band can slowly wear away at the stomach tissue. In severe cases, the wearing action of the band against the stomach can not only erode tissue, but also create a hole in the stomach, a serious complication that requires surgical repair.

Early band erosion occurs within the first six months after surgery and can appear within weeks of the procedure. Late band erosion appears at the six-month mark or after, so making it through the recovery phase is no guarantee that erosion will not occur. Regardless of when erosion happens, the news is not good for patients or their weight loss goals. The treatment for band erosion is typically surgical removal of the band appliance.

Symptoms of Gastric Erosion

Gastric erosion typically presents as bleeding that shows up in stool or vomit. Blood may make stool appear very dark or black in color, or it may take on a tarry appearance. Blood in the stool rarely looks red like what you may expect blood to look like. Blood may appear bright red when it appears in vomit, but it may also take on the appearance of coffee grounds.

In other cases, a patient may be diagnosed with anemia, which is a low red blood cell count. Erosion may be discovered during the process of determining what is causing the anemia, rather than because it is causing more obvious symptoms.

Diagnosing Band Erosion

The final diagnosis of band erosion typically requires endoscopy, a laparoscopic procedure that allows the surgeon to visualize the stomach through a tiny incision. A CT scan or an X-ray can also be beneficial in diagnosis.

Treatment of band erosion typically requires surgery and band removal to prevent further damage to the stomach.

Band Slipping

The gastric band is placed around the stomach in such a way that it makes a small pouch for food to be digested in before flowing through the band and through the digestive cycle. The lap band can move downward so that a greater portion of the stomach slips through the band, making the pouch larger. This allows a gastric banding patient to eat larger meals than intended. Doctors try to prevent slippage by using stitches to hold the band in the proper place, but this is not always successful.

Patients who eat meals larger than recommended and patients who vomit frequently are at the greatest risk for band slippage. If the band does move, it can be returned to its proper position, but doing so requires surgery.

SYMPTOMS OF A SLIPPED BAND:

- Rapid increase in reflux (heartburn)
- Sudden symptoms of an overly tight band
- Nausea and vomiting

Pouch Stretching

With many types of bariatric surgery, pouch stretching can be an issue. The stomach is a muscle, and can stretch over time, especially if larger meals than suggested are regularly eaten.

Concentric Pouch Dilatation

Concentric pouch dilation is a complication specific to gastric banding procedures. It happens when the band remains properly in place, but the pouch created stretches over time. This happens most often due to eating overly large meals repeatedly. Deflating the cuff temporarily may help improve the condition, but does not always prove an effective treatment. Severe cases may require band removal.

Deflating a Gastric Band Cuff

One of the benefits of the currently used gastric band appliances is that they are adjustable, meaning that they can be filled to provide greater restriction or released—emptied—to minimize the restriction. In some cases, where weight loss is of less importance than obtaining more calories, such as pregnancy or illness, the band can be temporarily released to allow larger meals to be consumed.

Long-Term Issues after Bypass Surgery

Gastric bypass procedures are most often a combination of a restrictive surgery, with all of the long-term issues those procedures present, and a bypass surgery, with the additional side effects caused by bypassing a portion of the intestine.

The good news is that bypass surgeries have the highest long-term success rate among bariatric surgeries. The not-so-good news is that they also have a higher risk of complications. This happens for two reasons. First, as with all surgeries, the more involved and extensive the procedure, the greater the risk. Second, decreasing the body's ability to absorb too many calories also works to decrease the amount of nutrients you can process.

Kidney Stones

Kidney stones, or renal calculi, are not uncommon after having bypass surgery. In fact, almost 10 percent of patients who have had gastric bypass experience at least one kidney stone within two years of having surgery.

SIGNS OF A KIDNEY STONE:

- Severe pain that comes in waves
- Blood in urine
- Painful urination
- Pain that increases after drinking
- Nausea and vomiting

The best way to prevent a kidney stone is to drink an adequate amount of water on a daily basis, taking in at least sixty-four ounces of water. Your calcium intake can also play a role in kidney stone formation, as too little calcium can increase the risk of forming stones. Conversely, too much Vitamin C and Vitamin D can contribute to the formation of stones. A diet high in sodium can also increase the chances of having a stone.

Unfortunately, a diet high in protein—one of the most important parts of the diet of any weight loss surgery patient—can also be a risk factor for kidney stones. A diet that is high in green, leafy vegetables, which are high in oxalate, will also increase the risk. Focusing on staying well-hydrated can often compensate for the high percentage of protein in the diet and help flush excess sodium from the body.

Malnutrition

Malnutrition is the lack of enough calories, or enough vitamins and minerals, to keep you healthy. Because the goal of surgery is to decrease the number of calories your body is able to utilize, it is important that every calorie you do absorb is nutrient rich. Eating a diet high in protein, typically a minimum of 60 grams per day, is essential to good health. In addition, fresh fruits and vegetables are high in vitamins in minerals, while low in fat and calories.

Focus on including at least one portion, even if it is a small one, of fresh fruit and fresh vegetables with most of your meals. Be sure to choose a wide variety of different colors of produce, as the rainbow of colors that are available also represent a wide range of nutrients that can prevent malnutrition.

ALERT

If your physician prescribes prescription-strength vitamin or mineral supplements, it is important that you do not take an over-the-counter supplement without first consulting your doctor. It is possible to get too much of a good thing, even essential nutrients!

After surgery, if you are low on vitamins and minerals, you are most likely to be low on iron and B vitamins. For that reason, prescription-strength supplements are typically part of daily life after weight loss surgery. While a diet rich in essential nutrients is of great importance after your procedure, it may not be enough to prevent iron deficiency or B vitamin deficiency, so be sure to take any supplements your surgeon recommends as directed.

One of the clearest signs of one type of malnutrition, vitamin (iron) deficiency anemia, is bruising easily. You may also feel fatigued, weak, and appear pale. If you are noticing these symptoms it is important to schedule an appointment with your physician to have some blood work done to test for anemia or another type of malnutrition complication.

If you have a condition that interferes with your ability to absorb nutrients, such as celiac disease, some liver and kidney conditions, or excessive alcohol consumption, your risk for malnutrition may be much higher.

Many physicians prescribe vitamin and mineral supplements to their patients who may be at risk for malnutrition. These prescriptions provide higher doses than can be found in over-the-counter supplements. If your doctor feels that you should be taking prescription-strength vitamins and minerals, it is essential that you take them as directed. Too few nutrients leads to malnutrition, but some can be harmful if too large a dose is taken. Never try to make up for a missed dose by taking two doses at the same time.

Osteoporosis

Osteoporosis is the medical term for weakened, fragile bone. Over time, osteoporosis can weaken bone so severely that a fall can lead to a broken hip or pelvis. Generally attributed to aging, and thought of as a disease of the elderly, it is a disease that can affect gastric bypass patients who are otherwise young and healthy. If your doctor suspects you are developing osteoporosis, a bone scan (a simple and painless procedure) may be done to determine the strength of your bones.

Preventing osteoporosis is far easier than treating it. One key component to preventing the disease from starting is to make sure that you have no less than 1,000 milligrams of calcium every day. While your diet should be rich in calcium, a supplement is recommended and can be purchased in most grocery stores. Your surgeon may recommend a dose that is higher than 1,000 milligrams per day, as your body may require a higher dose to obtain an adequate amount of calcium.

In addition to calcium supplements, weight-bearing exercise such as walking or aerobics can help strengthen and maintain bone mass.

Fat Soluble Vitamin Deficiency

Vitamins A, D, E, and K are fat-soluble vitamins, meaning that they are absorbed into the intestine along with fat molecules. They are also the most common vitamin deficiencies among gastric bypass patients. Gastric bypass makes it very difficult for the body to absorb these nutrients from food, making a supplement necessary.

To avoid vitamin deficiency, a supplement must be taken (commonly referred to as ADEK). Even with a supplement it is still important to eat fruits and vegetables rich in vitamins and nutrients. Vitamin A is commonly found in yellow and orange vegetables and fruits, especially sweet potatoes and carrots. Vitamin D is frequently added to milk, making vitamin D fortified skim milk an excellent source. Nuts and green fruits and vegetables such as kiwi, broccoli, and spinach are good sources of vitamin E. Vitamin K is found in green leafy vegetables such as spinach and kale, but it's also abundant in cabbage, cauliflower, and avocados.

Stenosis, Strictures, and Ulcers

An anastomosis is the surgical site where your surgeon reconnected your small intestine and parts of the stomach, depending upon the surgical procedure. While these incisions and suture lines are internal, they still have the potential to scar as much as your skin would, causing an abnormal narrowing in the area. This narrowing is referred to as stenosis, or a stricture. Over time, scar tissue and the healing process cause constriction in the tissue, making the area smaller. In the case of gastric bypass, narrowing happens where the anastomosis, or reconnection, is made.

The anastomosis that is done just past the stomach is referred as a stoma. This site is the most common place where scarring causes an abnormally small passageway for food. If the narrowing is severe, it can prevent food and even fluids from passing out of the stomach. This area is also susceptible to forming ulcers.

When severe narrowing occurs, surgery is required to open the area so that food and liquids can pass from the stomach into the intestine, or through the intestine, depending upon the surgical site affected.

Long-Term Issues for All Bariatric Patients

There are some long-term issues that all weight loss surgery patients face, regardless of the type of surgery that was performed. While some, such as an incision hernia, are a risk of any surgery that requires an incision, others are very specific to weight loss procedures.

Incisional Hernias

An incisional hernia occurs when an incision creates a weakness in a muscle, allowing the tissue underneath to push through the muscle toward the skin. The most common incisional hernias happen in the abdomen, where a small portion of tissue or even intestine pushed through the wall of the abdominal muscles. Laparoscopic, or minimally invasive, surgery typically decreases the risk of an incisional hernia, while an open procedure with the larger incision increases the risk.

An incisional hernia must be repaired surgically, but is not typically an urgent matter unless the tissue or organ that is pushing through the muscle is deprived of its blood supply. In that situation, the surgical repair is done on an emergency basis.

Too Much Weight Loss

It sounds like a dream come true in some ways, "Oh darn, I've lost too much weight!" But while it might sound wonderful, it can be a serious problem that takes major medical, and sometimes psychological help, to remedy. Being underweight can have many health consequences; much as obesity causes health problems, weighing too little can be a dramatic sign of malnutrition.

There are numerous conditions that can contribute to too much weight being lost, including anorexia and bulimia, an inability to absorb nutrients, chronic vomiting and diarrhea, and many more. Whether the cause is physical or psychological, intervention is required to remedy the situation.

In some cases, after being regimented about food intake for months or years, it can be difficult to eat enough to maintain a healthy weight. In this case, adding more fruits, vegetables, and whole grains to your diet can help you stop losing weight and maintain a healthy body size. Small additional portions can make a difference, without causing you to start gaining weight, erasing all that you've accomplished.

If you have trouble with too much weight loss, or have concerns about what your ideal weight truly is, speaking with your surgeon is a great way to clear up any questions you may have.

Pregnancy

Pregnancy is far more likely after you begin losing weight, as your fertility is likely to increase dramatically. However, for the sake of your total weight loss and the health of your child, you should avoid pregnancy for at least two years after your surgery, and even longer in some cases.

If you are a lap-band patient, it is possible to deflate your band completely to help you take in adequate nutrition, but with other types of surgery, it may be difficult to take in enough calories to support your body and that of a fetus.

Plan on taking measures to prevent pregnancy after your surgery, and consult with your surgeon if you do plan to become pregnant. Typically, once you've attained your goals, or are maintaining your weight loss, it is a safer time period to become pregnant. If you are considering having plastic surgery to remove excess skin, such as an abdominoplasty (tummy tuck), you may want to have the procedure after your pregnancy, as you may again end up with excess skin once you deliver.

Med Adjustments

One of the best side effects of weight loss surgery is that your other health conditions begin to improve as you lose weight in many cases. Patients who achieve significant weight loss often find that they are also losing conditions like type 2 diabetes, high blood pressure, and sleep apnea.

ESSENTIAL

If you are taking diabetes or high blood pressure medication and you begin to feel faint or lightheaded after your weight loss journey begins, you should see your doctor. One of the many potential causes for your symptoms is the dosage of your medication needing adjustment.

It is important that you don't quit your medications or try to adjust the doses yourself without speaking to your doctor. You may require more frequent visits to your primary physician in the months following surgery to adjust your medications as your blood sugar is more stable or your blood pressure is decreasing.

CHAPTER 4

Establishing and Meeting Your Goals

One of the big questions that patients ask before and after weight loss surgery is "how much weight will I lose?" Your surgeon will help you determine what a healthy and realistic goal is, but there are many types of goals and accomplishments after this type of procedure. Meeting your goals will require a great deal of time and effort, but it is well worth the effort, as your health and well-being will dramatically improve as the pounds come off.

Setting Realistic Goals

Medically speaking, weight loss surgery is considered successful if you lose 50 percent of your excess weight and you maintain that weight loss for a minimum of five years. That goal may or may not be appropriate for you. Many people are able to lose more than 50 percent of their excess weight and maintain that loss successfully. For some patients, meeting that 50 percent number is just not feasible or realistic.

One of the problems that patients face after surgery is separating realistic and not so realistic expectations. You may want to wear a size two and be able to wear a bikini, but wearing a size ten may be a much more likely outcome. The larger size is not a failure in any way and may represent a major achievement. A successful surgery does not mean that you will be skinny or wear a certain size of clothing, but there are still amazing rewards for weight loss. The goals you meet may not be in a clothing size, but in being able to stop taking prescription medication, or being able to go for a walk without being winded.

Patients who fall into the severe or super obese categories, with a BMI of 40 or greater, may still fall into the overweight or obese category after meeting their goals. This is not a failure, as it can represent weight loss of hundreds of pounds, and a vast improvement in health.

It is often difficult for patients to establish realistic weight loss goals for themselves. Your surgeon will be able to give you an idea of how much weight loss you can expect that takes into account the type of surgery, your current weight, age, and state of health, and many additional factors that affect weight. Your surgeon's idea of a goal weight may be far different from yours. She won't know what you weighed in high school, or how much you weighed when your husband proposed or what you considered your ideal weight in years past. Your surgeon will focus more on your body size and type, the outcomes that are typical after your procedure, and statistics about previous patients.

What Is a Reasonable Goal?

The medical community has agreed upon 50 percent of excess weight as a reasonable expectation for weight loss after surgery, but the reality is that there is no one single formula that can determine what amount of weight you can and will lose. The type of surgery you have is extremely important to your final result. Patients who have bypass surgeries often lose 70–80 percent of their excess weight, while 50 percent is much more likely for restrictive patients.

To calculate your excess weight:

1. Find a BMI chart that shows a grid of heights, weights, and a calculated BMI (Appendix A).
2. Find your current height and find the first weight column that shows a BMI of 25 or less. This will be your "normal weight."
3. Subtract your "normal weight" from your current weight. This is your excess weight.
4. Divide your excess weight in half.

This calculation gives you a rough estimate of the 50 percent weight loss that is considered adequate by the medical community.

How much weight you will lose is based on a variety of factors, and the surgery you selected will play a role in that, but the surgery is only one part of reaching your goal. Your adherence to your prescribed diet and the amount of exercise you incorporate into your daily routine will play a role that may prove to be just as important, if not more so.

Setting Goals Without a Scale

The amount of weight you would like to lose should be only one of your goals. There are many other things that your surgery should help you accomplish that aren't reflected on the scale. Try to consider your goal weight as just one small component of what you are trying to achieve. It is important to keep your goal weight in mind, but not to the exclusion of all of the other things you want to do as you shed pounds.

GOALS THAT AREN'T SET IN POUNDS:

- Climbing a flight of stairs without being out of breath
- Being able to run or walk for extended periods of time
- Having clothes that once were too small, becoming too big
- No longer needing diabetic medications

- Having normal blood pressure
- Working out five days a week
- Losing ten inches from your waist
- Sleep apnea no longer a problem
- Learning proper portion control
- No longer eating from boredom
- Removing junk food from your diet
- Trying a new sport or exercise
- Shopping at any clothing store, not a plus-size or "big" shop
- Having others notice your weight loss
- Fitting comfortably in a seat at the movies or on an airplane

Your goals may be more personal. Perhaps you want to be able to climb the stairs at work and reach your desk without huffing and puffing, or maybe there is a hill that you've decided you are going to conquer on your evening walk. Take the time to think about where you want to see improvements in your health and what you are able to accomplish physically, and incorporate those things into your goals.

Rewarding Yourself

What motivates you? Many people reward themselves with food, celebrating major and minor accomplishments and milestones with going to a restaurant or having dinner with friends. Finding ways to reward yourself after meeting a goal, getting good news, or accomplishing a task, is important to anyone who wants to lose weight. The challenge is to separate food from celebrating. Instead of going to dinner to celebrate a raise at work, would you feel rewarded if you had a massage instead? How about a night out while the kids are at home with a babysitter?

It is helpful to make a list of the things that truly motivate you to work harder, to stick with your goals, or just make you feel good. Then, you can pair short-term and long-term goals with different rewards. Did you go to the gym, work out for an hour, and stick to your diet 100 percent for the day? Time for a relaxing bubble bath with your favorite bath products. Do you love weekends in a bed and breakfast but think they are expensive and a real treat? That would be a great way to celebrate a major weight loss milestone. Have you always wanted to go to London, but never found the time? Think about using that as your reward when you reach your goal weight.

Your rewards do not need to be expensive to be effective, but they do need to be appropriate for your needs. Not everyone is motivated by the purchase of a new set of garden shears, just as some people are far from motivated by the idea of buying some new colors of nail polish. Think about what, other than a meal, makes you feel rewarded and start including those things in your celebrations.

If you struggle with one particular part of your weight loss plan, such as getting in enough exercise, or taking in enough fluids, those would be excellent accomplishments to acknowledge with your reward system. If working out feels more like plain old work, meeting your goal of working out five days per week should be acknowledged.

Five Keys to Success

A successful outcome after your surgery depends upon more than just what you eat. Of course your diet is essential to your success, but diet alone does not determine your final result. You may think that the only thing that matters is what you put in your mouth, but it truly is not that simple. In many ways your willingness to make exercise a regular part of your day, as well as learning to deal with your emotions and developing coping skills will be as important to your long-term weight maintenance as what you eat.

FIVE KEY COMPONENTS TO YOUR IMMEDIATE AND LONG-TERM SUCCESS:

1. Portion and calorie control
2. Exercise
3. Food choices
4. Emotional health
5. Accountability

Each of these elements play a role in getting to your ideal weight, but they will also help prevent something you may have experienced in the past: gaining back all the weight you have worked so hard to lose.

Portion and Calorie Control

Keeping your portion sizes under control and closely monitoring the total number of calories that you eat on a daily basis will form the foundation of your success. No weight loss surgery will have optimum results if your eating habits remain unchanged. Too many calories and too much food will undermine all of your other efforts to lose weight.

Portion and calorie control work hand in hand. It won't matter if your portions are the proper size if you are eating too many of them or if you are consuming too many calories. Controlling both the amount of food and the calorie content of your food will insure that your total food intake is appropriate for your needs.

Exercise

Exercise will do more than speed your weight loss, it will help you maintain your weight loss months and years after you reach your goal weight. Exercise will contribute to your improved health in many ways beyond burning calories. Weight-bearing exercise will help prevent osteoporosis, build muscle mass (which helps burn more calories!), and increase your energy level.

Food Choices

Your portion sizes may be in line, you may be consuming the right number of calories, but you could be headed for a serious case of malnutrition. The food you choose is just as important as the calories you consume, because every gram of protein and every vitamin and mineral count when you are on a diet reduced in volume.

For example, let's say you are able to consume 1,000 calories a day but you decide to eat five candy bars instead of balanced meals and snacks. You will be lacking in protein and essential nutrients, and you will be consuming a tremendous amount of fat and sugar. Every calorie you consume that is an empty calorie without nutritional value, such as sugar or junk food, takes the place of a calorie that could have been full of vitamins and minerals.

Emotional Health

If you truly want to have a successful long-term outcome you will have to deal with the emotional and psychological issues that led to your obesity in the first place. The vast majority of weight loss surgery patients have some sort of emotional eating that drives them to eat not when they are hungry, but for psychological reasons.

In many cases, food functions like a drug, soothing emotions and relieving stress. This effect often drives overeating, typically on an unconscious level. Have you ever been on a diet and doing great when something stressful happens? Something happens at work, or a relative is sick, or something of that nature, and you find yourself going off your diet and eating something sweet, salty, fatty, or maybe just eating far too much. This is an example of the type of behaviors you will have to identify and examine in order to stop eating emotionally and start eating to fuel your body.

Accountability

Taking control and responsibility for your weight loss and eating habits is a factor in both attaining your goals and maintaining them. No one can make you eat things that should not be present in your diet, no one will force you to eat a candy bar, or to skip a trip to the gym because you'd just rather not go. Taking personal responsibility for what you do to lose pounds and inches is key.

Your weight loss is exclusively under your control. There will always be the inevitable interruptions that prevent a workout or that require you to eat somewhere you'd prefer not to, but preparing for those issues and taking responsibility can make all the difference. If you know that you may have to stay late at work one day, and you will miss one of your workouts, taking responsibility means working out on a different day, or even going to the gym before work instead of after.

The mantra "I won't let anything stop me from reaching my fitness and weight loss goals" will help keep you on track and working to consistently improve your health. "I won't let _____ stop me from having a great day and meeting my goals, I will do _____ to make up for it" is one way of thinking about obstacles, then working around them.

Fitness Goals

Creating goals for fitness is a very personal thing. You may have no desire to start running, or you might have a condition that makes running a bad idea, so in that case to set a goal to run a marathon within two years of your surgery would not be appropriate. Perhaps you'd like to try yoga, or you love to swim but never do it because you don't like to wear a swimsuit in public. If that is the case, signing up for a yoga class, or feeling comfortable at a public pool are certainly appropriate goals.

Your fitness goals should strive to accomplish several things: to improve your physical strength, increase your stamina, help you reach your goal weight, and to incorporate exercise into your schedule on a regular basis. Meeting your goals will mean including more than one type of exercise into your program; both weight training, or using weights to strengthen your muscles, as well as aerobic activity should be part of your routine.

Getting Started on Day One

Starting your program won't wait until your recovery is over, it probably won't even wait for a full day after surgery. From the nurses getting you up and walking within hours of surgery, to the tiny meals you will have in the days following surgery, you will be on your program from the moment you leave the operating room.

Don't think that your weight loss plan will start a week or a month after you leave the hospital; it starts as soon as it possibly can. You may not be physically able to do a workout for a few weeks after surgery, but the expectation is that you do what you can as soon as you are able.

ESSENTIAL

Plan on walking the day of or the day after your surgery, increasing the amount of walking that you do each day after that. Your diet will be strictly limited initially, with the types of foods and the amount of food that you can take in increasing slowly over the course of the next weeks and months.

Each day is an opportunity to lose weight, and the first six months after your surgery will be when you can lose weight most easily. Don't waste the initial few weeks of that time waiting to get started after your recovery is over. This is also the best time to really focus on a high-quality diet, as the volume of food that you are able to consume will be very small, regardless of the type of surgery that you have.

Develop a Support System

A support system is essential to your emotional well-being as you go through the major changes that surgery will start. Identify people in your life that you can count on to be there when you need them, whether as a workout buddy, a shoulder to cry on, or just someone who doesn't mind listening as you work on improving your health.

Success comes much easier when you work as a team, and while you are ultimately responsible for your weight loss, it is always a good thing to have people who are willing to be your own personal cheerleaders. Perhaps you have a friend who is outrageously upbeat and positive, a great person to talk to when you're feeling down. A friend who exercises religiously may be the ideal person to be a workout buddy, someone who will call to remind you that you have an exercise date or to see if you'd like to go for a walk.

Different people are able to be supportive in different ways. A friend who loves to cook and has hundreds of cookbooks may be able to help you create new recipes that meet your dietary restrictions.

Your friends, coworkers, and family members may all have something to offer, and you may find support in places you didn't expect. Your church may have a walking or workout program that you never even considered joining; your neighbor may enjoy some company on those nightly excursions when she walks her dog. Look for opportunities to be supported and encouraged or to have company while you work toward your goals.

Are You Open or Private about Surgery?

While thinking about your support system, you may realize that you are not sure how willing you are to share your journey. Are you the kind of person who doesn't care if everyone at work, church, the PTA, and the gym knows that you've had weight loss surgery? Or are you more private, feeling that surgery is a very personal decision and no one's business but your own and whomever you may decide to tell? The decision is entirely your own. Most people fall somewhere in the middle, not broadcasting the information, but willing to talk about it if someone asks.

Sharing the information freely has benefits and drawbacks, just as keeping the information private does. If you choose to share the information, you may find that you receive support from people you may have never expected to be part of your personal cheerleading squad. That health nut at work who walks for an hour at lunchtime may just be willing to have you join in the fun! You may also find that people you would have never suspected of having weight loss surgery, because they are thin and healthy, are actually weight loss surgery patients themselves, and have valuable advice and guidance to offer. If you don't share the fact that you've had surgery, you may not realize these resources are available because they won't have as many opportunities to present themselves.

On the other hand, keeping the information private is a very positive. thing in some ways. Most weight loss surgery patients have had the experience where an acquaintance has said something like "Why did you have surgery? That is taking the easy way out; all you needed to do was eat less and get off of the couch once in a while." While this statement is wrong on many levels, you may not hear it as often if you are less open about your procedure.

Whatever you decide to say or not say about your surgery, at some point it will be completely obvious that you've shed a great number of pounds. Coworkers, friends, and even relatives are bound to have questions about how you've done so well, and it is fair to say that you've radically changed your diet and started exercising, even if that isn't the entire truth.

Avoiding Saboteurs

If you've ever been on a diet, you've probably already had the diet saboteur experience. They come in many forms: the coworker who knows you are on a diet but tries to talk you into going to dinner anyway; the family member who brings a giant version of your favorite cake over on your birthday; or the person who says you look fantastic the way you are and tries to get you to return to your old habits.

Some saboteurs are more toxic than others. It is usually obvious who is well-meaning and doesn't mean to harm your diet versus the manipulative type who will attempt to derail your success. There are many reasons why someone would want to stop your weight loss, even though it means damaging your health and quality of life. Your spouse may feel that if you are thin, you may want a divorce; your friend may prefer to be the "pretty one" while you remain the "fat one." You may experience others who are just threatened when someone else succeeds where they have failed. "Just this one time won't hurt" is a common quote from people who aren't putting your best interests first.

Dealing with Saboteurs

You may already have an idea of who may try to undermine your efforts, whether it is the aunt who is a fantastic cook or the boss who has been dieting unsuccessfully for the last ten years. In most cases, you won't have to avoid these people; you'll just want to avoid eating with them. Concerned that your friend is jealous of your success? Don't talk about it in her presence and be vague when asked questions about your weight loss.

ESSENTIAL

Going to a family celebration where you know that someone will try to tempt you into eating something you shouldn't or something that will make you sick, like a sugar-laden dessert? Go to the function after having a full meal, or better yet, take a dish that fulfills your nutritional needs and eat with the family, secure in the knowledge that you are staying on your plan.

The key to success when dealing with people who will derail your efforts is to identify them before they do damage to your diet. If someone has the potential to hurt your results, be honest with them. The vast majority of people don't mean to cause you harm, and, if you approach them in a gentle way, will typically change their behavior. Saying something like, "I know we used to go to lunch on a regular basis, but I can no longer do that and I really need your support on this to be successful," can often be the key to converting a saboteur into a support person.

Each Day Is a New Day

No one is perfect, as the saying goes, and that includes you, regardless of how much you might want to be absolutely perfect with your weight loss plan. The key is not letting a single slip lead to a full day's, week's, or month's worth of slips. One overly large meal does not make you a failure, but making sure it doesn't become routine will make an enormous difference in your final result.

Each morning is a new opportunity to have a day that positively impacts your goals. It is a fresh start where you can hop out of bed knowing that you will eat the right things and make the time to exercise. This is your opportunity to plan for a great day; packing your lunch with nutritious food, rather than eating fast food because it was the only option available to you; or making sure your gym bag has everything you need in it so you have no excuses for avoiding the treadmill.

Learning from a Bad Day

Take a bad day and make it a learning experience. If you were tempted to overeat, what led to that feeling? Were you feeling sad, stressed, bored, or any other emotions that may have triggered the episode? In many twelve-step programs addicts are taught that there are four feelings that are highly likely to trigger a "drug binge" whether that drug is food, sex, illicit drugs, or something else. Those emotions are hunger, anger, loneliness, and feeling tired. If you are feeling any of those things, and are tempted to self-medicate with food, stop, take a deep breath, and decide how you are going to deal with the feeling in a positive manner. Frequently, being aware that a trigger is present is enough to allow you to cope in a positive way, rather than doing something that you will later regret. Your food diary, if you include how you were feeling when you ate each meal, may help reveal patterns of behavior that affect your eating habits.

CHAPTER 5

The First Six Months

t six months after your weight loss procedure will
exciting and challenging. You can expect to face
nanges in your lifestyle and eating habits and most
nt, you will be developing new habits and coping
hile this time won't be easy, your hard work will be
d with better health and significant weight loss.

Your Golden Opportunity

The first six months after your surgery is truly your golden opportunity. This is the time when your weight loss will be the most dramatic, and when you will make radical changes to your lifestyle.

Your willingness to change how you eat, start exercising, and work at understanding why you are prone to overeating will determine how successful you are immediately after surgery and in the years following. A general rule of thumb for your weight loss is that you will realize half of your overall weight loss in the first six months, then a similar amount in the following year. The amount you lose in the first six months plays a huge role in determining your final weight and whether you will meet your weight loss goals.

ALERT

While your surgery will certainly make it easier for you to lose weight, it is not a magic pill. Surgery is one piece of a four-part approach that also includes understanding the emotional part of overeating, nutritional changes, and exercise. Ignoring any one of these four basic components can mean that you will not be as successful.

Secrets of Successful Weight Loss Patients

People who lose weight successfully have many things in common that help them meet and maintain their goals. The big thing they share is the fact that they never gave up, even after having a bad diet day or skipping too many days of exercise. They kept working toward their goal. That perseverance, day after day, slowly but surely led to weight loss success.

MORE HABITS OF SUCCESSFUL WEIGHT LOSS PATIENTS:

- Make exercise part of each day.
- Incorporate weight training into your exercise program.
- Keep a food diary.
- Make your goal "being healthy," not a particular weight or size.
- Eat slowly.

- Stop eating impulsively.
- Wait for "stomach hunger," not a particular time of day

Expect the Unexpected

Many people underestimate the overall effects of surgery on their lives, both physically and emotionally. It can't be emphasized enough that problems and complications can arise after surgery, and often do. Sometimes these issues are minor, such as difficulty eating in the weeks following surgery, and in other cases the problems are more significant, such as marital problems that arise as weight loss boosts self-confidence and independence.

There will be a tremendous number of positive changes that are worth celebrating after your surgery. Fitting into smaller sizes and watching the number on the scale move downward are worth celebrating. Improving overall health is also a major benefit of weight loss. However, those rewards will not come without sacrifice and may be very stressful.

Eating May Be Difficult

In the initial weeks following your surgery, you may want to eat and even be encouraged to eat more, but you cannot. Your body may not be happy with even the smallest morsels of food, and you may struggle to find something that you are able to eat. While on the surface this is great for weight loss, it can be a very difficult time and very stressful.

It may take weeks or even longer to be able to follow your surgeon's recommendations on what you should be eating and how much. It is important that you keep in contact with your surgeon regarding your inability to eat, or if you are only able to eat far less food than is recommended.

For most people, issues with being able to eat resolve on their own, and you will be able to take increasingly large meals over time. While you will never be able to eat the volume of food that you were able to consume prior to surgery, you should be able to eat a healthful amount of food.

Complications Can Happen

Prior to your surgery your physician discussed the possible complications of surgery with you. It may have seemed like a laundry list of problems, ranging from blood clots to hernias and even including death. Many patients have the attitude that complications happen to other patients, not to them. But the majority of surgery patients will face some type of complication, albeit typically minor ones.

FACT

Make sure your surgeon is aware of all of the medications you are taking, both prescription and over the counter, as well as any medical conditions you may have. You may be predisposed to certain kinds of complications that may be easily prevented.

During your recovery from surgery and even months or years later, you should be on the lookout for problems that may be related to your surgery. You will need to be proactive; if you are at risk for osteoporosis and other malnutrition problems, you may even need to request lab tests from your physician that will determine if you need vitamin supplements.

The key to managing complications is to spot them before they become serious. Be assertive in seeking answers and treatment if you feel something is wrong. If you are feeling tired and lethargic all the time, don't assume it is just because you are exercising more; you could be anemic or you could be lacking in essential vitamins and nutrients. You will also need to keep a close eye on any conditions you had prior to surgery. For example, people who are diabetic will need to monitor their blood glucose closely, as medication needs can change radically with weight loss.

Relationships Change

Expect your relationships with friends, family, and coworkers to change. This can be aggravating, hurtful, and even shocking, but your weight loss will cause changes in the way you relate with people that may be unexpected. Many find that they didn't realize they were being treated badly due to their weight until they were no longer heavy. Others find that friends drift away, jealous or uncomfortable with the radical changes brought about by weight loss.

Many weight loss surgery patients find that they feel more assertive and confident as the weight comes off. As self-esteem improves, many find that they will no longer tolerate certain behaviors from loved ones. Sometimes a spouse may feel as though the person he or she married is no longer there, replaced by a thin person who seems like a stranger.

Support groups and therapy, including marriage counseling, can be of great benefit when relationships are being affected by a radical change in weight and the subsequent emotional changes.

Maximizing Your Results

Eat less, exercise more, and lose lots of weight, right? Well, if it were that simple, you would have done it without surgery! Maximizing your weight loss is hard work, and while it does include eating less and working out more, that is an overly simplified look at weight loss.

You will be eating less calories than you did prior to surgery, and you will need to exercise to be successful, but those things can be difficult. Over time you will develop tools that help you to be successful, such as keeping tempting foods out of your cupboards, finding activities to replace eating when feeling stressed, and strategies for eating in restaurants.

While the key to weight loss is consuming less calories and burning more, developing ways to do both long term are key. Making a lifetime change will take time and diligent work. Many people have stuck with a diet for a few weeks or months, but the goal here is to make changes that can be maintained for life.

ALERT

Soda and other beverages can seriously derail your weight loss efforts. Just one soda a day can add up to over 62,000 calories in your diet over a year. That's eighteen pounds not lost!

Therapy and Support Groups

While many feel that support groups and therapy are not for them, won't help, or are just silly, research is showing that patients who participate have better outcomes. They are better equipped to deal with challenges, experience positive peer pressure from their support group, and make the effort to determine what is emotionally driving their overeating. Certainly a therapist isn't required to accomplish these things, but there are a multitude of reasons why therapy and support groups are strongly recommended before and after surgery.

Seeking support from someone outside your circle of family and friends can be very beneficial. Support groups for weight loss surgery patients are great for sharing your struggle, sharing your concerns and issues with others, and learning coping tools from your peers.

Therapy, which is one-on-one counseling, or may involve couples counseling, can also be beneficial. It may be helpful to find a therapist who has experience with weight loss surgery patients, or who specializes in helping those who have issues with overeating.

Nutrition and Calories

Part of successfully losing weight is learning about your nutritional needs. You will need to know the number of calories you should consume each day, how to choose nutritionally dense foods, and much more. Over time you will include more fresh fruits and vegetables in your diet and eliminate processed foods that are high in calories but mostly devoid of vitamins and minerals. Lean proteins, such as chicken, pork, and dairy, will play a large role in your diet.

Tips for Portion Control

If you struggle with the smaller portion sizes that are appropriate after weight loss surgery, you are not alone. Consider some of these strategies to make less food feel like more:

- In a restaurant, immediately place any food that is over a proper portion size in a to-go container.
- Use smaller plates, to make your plate look full.
- Start your meal with a low-calorie broth or salad.
- If you don't feel satisfied and want another serving, wait five minutes then decide.
- Chew your food slowly and thoroughly.

- Put your fork down between bites; this will help you slow down and savor your food.
- Don't wait until you are starving to eat.
- Have a large glass of water half an hour before you eat.

Learn to Cook Healthy Meals

You may be an accomplished cook, but more than likely you will need to adjust both how and what you cook. Cooking for yourself is the best way to control what you eat, allowing you to closely monitor calories, portion size, and nutritional content. Cooking your own meals can be time consuming, but it will greatly improve your chances of meeting your goal weight, as most restaurants serve overly large portions that are high in fat and calories.

You may need to learn new cooking techniques and recipes in order to meet your dietary needs. Your old favorites might not be appropriate for everyday meals and may need to be reserved for special occasions. There are also common habits that you may need to break, such as frying foods or sautéing in butter.

Your new focus will be on fresh and lean foods that are high in vitamins and minerals and full of protein and fiber. Fat is a source of flavor, so you will be replacing the flavor that is "missing" by seasoning your food well and using methods that add flavor without adding substantial calories.

ESSENTIAL

After your surgery, you will want to focus on methods of cooking that don't add calories or fat to your meal. This is easier than it sounds, as you probably are already familiar with the most common ways to cook without butter and oil: baking, broiling, grilling, steaming, and poaching.

Changing Tastes

The good news about changing the way you cook is that your taste in food will change rather quickly. It may be hard to believe, but after a few short weeks eating a low-fat diet, fatty foods will taste greasy and oily, and will not be as appealing as they once were. The same is true of sodium.

Food that once tasted properly seasoned will taste overly salty once you remove excess sodium from your diet for as little as a week or two.

In time, freshly steamed vegetables will taste great, and vegetables that are overcooked or dressed with butter and sauces will no longer be appealing. They may look wonderful, and they may be the source of cravings, but your first bite will be a disappointment.

Embracing Exercise

Exercise is the best tool for boosting weight loss, improving personal appearance, and maintaining your goal weight. Not only does exercise burn calories, it also increases your metabolism, tones muscle, and improves cardiovascular fitness. It's also a great way to compensate for a larger than normal meal, or to make sure that a holiday meal doesn't result in weight gain.

Once you've lost weight, your need for exercise will not change, as it will be the way you maintain your weight loss and keep your body slim. It will get easier though, as you become accustomed to working out and your body fat is decreased. Just think about how much easier it will be to walk a mile when your body is a hundred pounds lighter!

Exercise Doesn't Have to Be Work

Making exercise fun, or at least less like work, will help you create and maintain an exercise program. You do not have to walk on a treadmill for thirty minutes every day to be successful. If you like that, certainly do it, but feel free to mix it up with aerobics classes, biking, swimming, team sports, hiking, and many other activities that will get your heart pumping. Don't hesitate to add music to your workout to help you keep your pace up, or watch your favorite television program to make the time pass more quickly.

Working on the Inside

One of the most important things you will do after your surgery is identify the emotions and situations that trigger food cravings and overeating. You will also need to explore what has led to overeating in the past, as a way to prevent it in the future.

Surgery alone won't fix your desire to overeat. You will need to determine what motivates the way you eat so that you can change your pattern of behavior. As you learn more about what causes you to eat for emotional reasons, rather than for nutrition, you will learn ways to cope with those feelings.

Eating Out of Boredom

Eating out of boredom is a common problem that can derail weight loss. You may find yourself wandering into the kitchen not because you are hungry, but just to occupy your time. If you find yourself reaching for a snack, take the time to think about whether you need a snack, or if you are just eating because it is there.

Unconscious Eating

Unconscious eating, or eating without paying attention, is a similar problem that can also stop weight loss. A great example is eating popcorn at a movie theater; you may find that you reach the bottom of the bucket without remembering eating most of it, or even enjoying it.

Plan on eating consciously, paying attention to what you are eating and how you feel while eating—chewing slowly, waiting for the physical sensation of fullness, then stopping. It may be helpful to eat all of your meals while sitting at a table rather than in front of the television or computer.

Depression

Many people use food to self-medicate when they are feeling depressed. It may be a fleeting feeling of being down or a more chronic problem with depression that triggers the need to eat. The body actually responds to eating carbohydrates by producing serotonin, the chemical that gives us pleasure and combats depression, so self-medicating can develop out of a need to feel better.

If you find that you are feeling blue and it triggers eating, you will want to find another way to combat the feeling. Exercise is a great way to feel better and avoid eating, but if the feelings of depression linger, you may want to seek medication or treatment from your physician.

Some weight loss surgery patients actually feel more depressed after surgery, because they are no longer treating the symptoms with food. Identifying these feelings and the resulting urge to eat is the first step, but finding a way to cope with the depression is essential.

Feeling Like an Outsider

Some patients report feeling like an outsider after their procedure. For some this is caused by eating a liquid diet and tiny portions while everyone else is going to lunch. Others have difficulty watching loved ones overeat, and they feel like they are the only person they know who isn't consuming too much food.

In some cases, the radical change in lifestyle makes people feel like they no longer have much in common with their friends, or their children are resentful because junk food and fatty meals are no longer part of the household. These issues are normal after surgery, but while frustrating, they cannot be allowed to derail your plans, goals, and ultimately, your success.

Weight Loss Will Not Make Your Problems Go Away

It is easy to imagine that life as a thin person will be better. It will be better in many ways, but your life won't suddenly become perfect. The problems that you faced prior to surgery will not suddenly disappear, and new problems will be caused by the changes you are experiencing.

While some problems certainly can be solved by the surgery, such as hypertension or type 2 diabetes, surgery won't improve your financial problems or disagreements with your teenager. Your spouse won't suddenly do his or her fair share of the housework because of your procedure, and your job won't become less tedious. Enjoy the benefits of your surgery, but don't count on surgery to improve everything.

Twenty Tips for Success

Here are twenty things you can do to put yourself on the right road toward success.

1. Avoid drinking calories.
2. Exercise every day, even if just for a few minutes.
3. Keep a food diary.
4. Find a support group.
5. Drink at least sixty-four ounces of water per day.
6. Keep your appointments with your doctors.
7. Don't weigh yourself too frequently.
8. Take your measurements regularly.
9. Make your exercise as pleasant as possible by reading a book, listening to music, or exercising with friends.
10. Don't drink fluids half an hour before or after a meal.
11. Follow your surgeon's instructions to the letter.
12. Look for ways to include exercise in your day, such as taking the stairs.
13. Don't keep trigger foods in the house.
14. Before taking a single bite, ask yourself if you are "stomach hungry" or "head hungry."
15. Focus on eating the protein serving before eating the rest of your meal.
16. Don't expect perfection, but do plan for it.
17. Find exercises that you enjoy, not just the ones that burn the most calories.
18. Measure your food; don't assume your portion sizes are correct.
19. Accept the support offered by friends and family.
20. Reward yourself frequently for your accomplishments and hard work.

CHAPTER 6

Emotional Issues after Weight Loss Surgery

After you have surgery there will be few, if any, areas of your life that are not changed by your dramatic weight loss. In addition to the alterations in your relationship with food, your relationships with friends and family will be altered. The way you approach meals and social gatherings will change, and you may be distressed to find that your weight loss seems to be causing changes in other people.

Coping with Change

The first few months after your surgery will be full of change. You will be making massive changes to your diet, you will be exercising regularly, and you will be focused on your nutritional habits in a way you probably never have been in the past. It seems straightforward, but those changes will be far more emotional than you can probably imagine before surgery.

You may think that your life will be the same other than at meal times, or that all of the changes in your life will be positive. Many people believe that if they just lose weight their lives will be perfect. In fact, losing weight can create more issues than it solves, and may make you far more aware of problems you may have dismissed or ignored in the past.

Don't misunderstand, weight loss surgery, and the subsequent weight loss itself, is a wonderful thing. You will be healthier, you will look better, and you will have far more energy than you did in the past. You may have health issues that completely resolve as the pounds come off, and you may find that any chronic pain you have, from your feet to your back, is greatly improved.

With all of those positive physical changes come emotional changes and issues that can complicate and change your life. Many of the changes will be very positive in nature, but there can be unexpected complications in your life as well.

Other Areas of Your Life Will Change

It is hard to imagine that something as straightforward as losing weight will change many facets of your life, but it will. Some changes may be smaller, such as how you dress and the types of clothing that you prefer. Other changes will be much greater, including changes in what you find acceptable behavior in others, what you like to do in your free time, and how you interact with your children. You may find yourself feeling the need for more independence and starting to do things you never would have considered in the past.

These changes may be largely positive, but it is important to be aware that sweeping changes throughout your life are coming. The hard work you will be doing physically and emotionally will have a dramatic impact on how you see your life and what you want and need for yourself. You may find that you develop a different group of friends or that you have the courage to make major life changes that seemed impossible prior to surgery.

Losing the "Comfort" of Food

Many people have the realization that they have a problem with food immediately after surgery, when they are eating as little as a tablespoon of food at a time. When you are physically unable to eat or are eating very little, it can become shockingly apparent how much you use food in response to stress or moods, rather than for nutrition.

ESSENTIAL

There may be many different moments of realization, when the overwhelming desire or need to eat something sweet or salty, or a comfort food, is obviously not "stomach hunger." Learning to eat when your body is hungry, rather than for emotional reasons (head hunger) can be very challenging and can require counseling and therapy.

When you go from eating whatever you want, and enough of it to maintain a morbidly obese body weight, to a strictly controlled low-calorie diet, it can be very difficult. While your surgery can help prevent overeating, the most important thing is getting to the root of what drives you to overeat. What feelings are you trying to squelch or soothe when you think about reaching for a piece of chocolate or some potato chips?

If you are an emotional eater, eating in times of stress and unhappiness, it may be very uncomfortable to avoid food when you would have "self-medicated" with food in the past. Some surgery patients report bursting into tears when they get home after a stressful day, head to the kitchen, and realize that they cannot use food to cope with what they are feeling. Others report feelings of depression when they cannot use food as a coping mechanism.

Head Hunger versus Stomach Hunger

Head hunger is just what it sounds like; a need to eat not based on a physical need, but from stress, emotions, or other feelings that happen in your head. Stomach hunger is the actual physical need to eat; a growling stomach, feeling hungry out of a need to fuel the body.

If you have reached the point of obesity, it is very likely that your eating habits are more in tune with head hunger than stomach hunger. You may have even learned to ignore your body's cues to eat or to stop eating. Conquering the desire to eat for emotional reasons will be one of the most important things you can do to lose weight and keep it off.

Surgery does not change your emotional relationship with food. It may remind you to stop eating after a reasonable amount of food, but surgery cannot do the hard work of getting to the bottom of what drives you to overeat. If you are experiencing these feelings of "needing" to eat even though your body is satiated, consider writing down exactly what triggered the feeling, how you reacted with a food craving, and what you did to conquer the feeling in a healthy manner.

Many people require therapy or a support group to truly understand what is driving them emotionally to overeat, and to establish coping skills that do not include food.

Body Image and Self-Esteem

After experiencing weight loss, it is natural to feel a dramatic improvement in your self-esteem and feelings of self-worth. In many ways, obese people are made to feel like they are less attractive and less valuable than their thinner counterparts. That can be true at home, in the workplace, and in social situations.

As you continue to lose weight and fit in the more stereotypical ideal of beauty, others will certainly begin to be complimentary, even if you aren't feeling the boost in your body image yet. The compliments may help you develop better feelings about yourself and your appearance, but you may find that working hard and finding success is equally important.

As you continue to lose weight and exercise, you will experience a variety of feelings about your body and your personal appearance. You will have the emotional high of shopping in new stores and for sizes you haven't worn for years, but you will also have to deal with family and even friends telling you that you are too thin.

What Happened to My Body?

When you start the weight loss process, you may imagine that you will have an amazing body at the end of the process. While you will certainly be much thinner, you may find that your body doesn't look exactly the way you expected it to. You may have excess skin that hangs loose from your body; if you are female you may find that your breasts look very different than they did before surgery. While some of these changes will improve over time and with exercise, your excess skin may require plastic surgery.

Will I Ever Be Happy with My Body?

You may have disliked or even hated your body when you were obese, but you still aren't happy with your body now that you have lost large amounts of weight. This may lead you to wonder if you will ever be happy with what you see in the mirror. The truth is pretty simple—maybe.

You may never learn to love your body, but liking your body is a process. It means not comparing your body to images you see in fashion magazines or on television. Liking your body means being happy about the things that make you unique, appreciating your good health, and making an effort to take good care of yourself.

FACT

Body Dysmorphic Disorder, or BDD, is a condition where a person becomes overly concerned, or even obsessed, about what they view as a flawed body part. It can occur as some weight loss patients reach their goal weight, but still see a morbidly obese person in the mirror. Others may pursue plastic surgery to correct physical flaws that they feel are severe, but are not notable to others.

Liking your body can be as simple as saying to yourself "I like my body" as often as you need to, until you absolutely believe it. It can also be as complicated as requiring psychological therapy and even some plastic surgery to take care of post-surgery issues that are present after you reach your goal. Regardless of how you reach the point of liking your body, being content in your own skin is a priceless gift you give yourself.

Finding Support

One of the best things you can do for yourself after surgery is create a strong support system. You will need to have people you can talk to about your experience with surgery, what you are feeling as you lose weight, and all of the emotions that come along with making sweeping changes in your lifestyle.

You may be pleasantly surprised to find that different people are able to provide support and encouragement in different ways. You may have a friend who has been through the surgery and can provide guidance and an understanding of what you are living. You may have another friend who is a fantastic cook, who can provide support in the form of recipes and cooking help.

FACT

Support takes many forms. A friend who is willing to chat and make small talk on the phone can be very valuable when you are trying to distract yourself from raiding the fridge. Don't discount the friends who are happy to hear from you but who don't necessarily know anything about weight loss or your surgery.

Friends and Family

Friends and family are the most obvious choices for an informal support group, as they are probably the people who know you best. You may find that they are a great resource, listening while you talk about the difficulties and changes you are experiencing.

That said, friends and family may also say things like "do you talk about anything other than losing weight?" If they haven't walked in your shoes, being overweight and doing the work of losing a tremendous amount of weight, they may not understand how consuming it can be. If you are able to rely on those closest to you for the support you need, fantastic, but you may also want to look for people who have been through surgery who can completely empathize with what you are going through.

Weight Loss Surgery Support Groups

Support groups are a great way to find people who completely understand what you are experiencing because they have been through it themselves. These groups are often sponsored by surgery clinics or by surgeons, encouraging patients to support each other through the process. These groups have benefits outside of psychological support, as they can also be a great place to exchange clothing as you rapidly change sizes, trade recipes, and even find a workout buddy.

Don't underestimate the power of sharing the experience of weight loss. These groups are designed to be supportive but also to help you hold yourself accountable for what you are doing to lose weight. If you know you will be meeting with your group, you may find a little more willpower to resist that food you know you shouldn't eat, because you know you will be surrounded by people who are facing the same challenges.

Online Support

If you are too far away from a support group meeting, or feel that the meetings aren't for you, consider joining an online support group. There are dozens of places on the Internet where you can meet and talk with others about your shared experience. There are question-and-answer forums, places where you can chat, and even more formal meetings with a set day and time for meetings.

Therapy

You may find yourself saying that you don't need therapy, or that therapy is for people with serious mental health issues or other major problems. Don't be too quick to remove the possibility of seeking therapy from your options. Many people who have reached and maintained their goal weight credit therapy for helping them do it.

Therapy, especially one-on-one therapy, can be a great way to get to the bottom of the emotional issues that contributed to your obesity in the first place. A good therapist can also help you find ways to effectively cope, instead of overeating. There are therapists who specialize in caring for people after weight loss surgery, who are familiar with the issues that you are facing now and may have in the future. In fact, many surgeons actually have a therapist on staff, or one they frequently recommend, to help their patients.

I'm Losing Weight—Why Is Everyone Else So Different?

In the course of your weight loss you may find that you are treated differently than before. People who didn't speak to you before now seek you out for conversation; people you were close to seem to pull away from you. This is a common experience among people who lose large amounts of weight.

While in many ways you may feel like you are the same person you always were, the major changes in your body are evident to those around you and will lead to people looking at you in new and different ways.

These changes can be very positive. The women who walk during their lunch hour at work may invite you to participate. You may make new friends at the gym and during exercise sessions that you didn't participate in prior to your surgery. You may find yourself feeling more outgoing, so you find yourself speaking to people you may not have in the past. Along with those positive things, you may find that people you thought you could count on for support are no longer among your closest friends, and others don't seem to share your joy at what you've accomplished.

I'm a New Person!

You may feel like a brand new person as you slip into smaller sizes. You may feel more sociable and confident, and your self-esteem may be greatly improved. There are so many positive things going on, you may feel like you are becoming a new person on the inside and the outside.

As you are feeling like a new person, the people around you may insist on treating you as though nothing has changed. They may still want to go out and grab drinks after work or an ice cream after lunch. Your family may still expect you to make fatty meals or foods that are not part of your diet plan. Your friends may be disappointed that you no longer bring baked goods to social functions.

There may be days when you want to scream from the rooftops that you've changed. You no longer overeat and you don't focus on food like you once did. It can be very frustrating when people expect you to be like you used to be, when you've made such positive changes in your life.

ESSENTIAL

You may find that in many ways you are the same person, with the same problems, concerns, and issues you had prior to surgery and weight loss, but you are also a totally different person, with new habits, new goals, and an entirely new appearance. Feeling pulled between who you were, who you are, and who you are becoming is a very normal feeling after weight loss surgery.

You may actually have to say, "I'm no longer able to do those things, so perhaps we could come up with an alternative" when people continue to try to push you back into your old habits. Don't allow anyone to make you feel guilty for making changes in your life that lead to much better health.

I'm the Same Person I Was 100 Pounds Ago!

While part of you may be thinking "I'm a brand new person," there is another side to the same coin . . . the part of you that is very much the same. It can be very difficult to tolerate people who knew you before surgery treating you as though you are better or smarter or more interesting simply because you've lost weight.

It can be very frustrating to have people treat you differently, when you are essentially the same person you were before. It's a difficult balance; in many ways you want people to realize you've made huge changes in your life and you want people to respect the choices you've made, but you don't want to be treated differently just because you are thinner. It can be hard to find a balance; having family and friends respect the alterations you've made in your diet but realize that you are essentially the same inside, despite the outer differences.

Now I Am Angry!

Some successful dieters experience anger as they move along their weight loss journey. The anger stems from one simple but sad fact: Obese people are treated differently by society as a whole. Even if absolutely nothing changes about you but your clothing size, you will be treated differently. Studies have shown that overweight people have a harder time finding good jobs and experience a variety of forms of discrimination, whether they realize it or not.

It can be a difficult thing to find out how you have been treated just because of the way you look. You may want to discuss it with your support group, as they will have their own experiences to share. You aren't alone in feeling that you are treated differently as a thin person, but you cannot allow your anger over the situation to derail your success.

When Good Friends Turn Bad

While most friends and family just want you to be happy and healthy, you may have people in your life who aren't as happy for you as you might have expected. In fact, they seem downright bitter, angry, or even jealous about what you are doing. You may hear critical comments meant to downplay your success, or outright negativity regarding what you've accomplished.

If someone you consider a friend is trying to belittle your weight loss, or even worse, trying to sabotage your success, you will have to put a stop to it. Hopefully, a frank conversation where you request their assistance with your progress and an end to the negativity will do the trick, but in some cases your success will mean the end of a friendship.

The Food Police

There are many people who think that knowing that you had a weight loss procedure gives them a license to comment on everything you eat. They may encourage you to eat more, since you are obviously starving yourself, or they may act as though you have committed a crime if they see you eating a Christmas cookie.

Don't be temped to eat more just because other people believe you aren't eating enough. You know what you should be eating, and what a proper portion size is for you. Don't let outside influences alter your meal plans.

Many people will weigh in on what you are eating, how much you are eating, and whether or not you should be eating it. Just keep your goal in mind and eat what you know is right for you. If you decide to indulge in a treat, compensate for it by reducing calories in other areas or exercising more, and don't worry about the comments of others.

Weight Loss Is Not a Magic Happiness Pill

When people have weight loss surgery, they often have the belief that life will be wonderful after surgery. While being thin is a wonderful thing, it doesn't mean that your life will be perfect. It is not abnormal to find that losing weight creates almost as many problems as it solves.

More Attention

Don't be surprised if you attract more attention, both positive and negative, than you have in the past. It is an unfortunate fact that many people will be jealous or resentful of your accomplishments, and you will be treated differently by people who have known you for years.

You may find yourself receiving far more attention from the opposite sex than you have in the past, even from people who seemed to ignore you before surgery. While you may be the same person on the inside, the outside is changing dramatically and people will notice.

You may enjoy the added attention, especially if dating more or meeting someone was one of the things that motivated you to lose weight, or you might find the attention unwanted.

Marriage and Divorce

If your motivation for having weight loss surgery included improving your marriage, you may be shocked to find that there is a higher rate of divorce among those who have the surgery than those who do not. There are a variety of reasons for the statistic, including the heightened self-esteem of the spouse that lost weight, a change in how independent one spouse is, and, commonly, a spouse that doesn't know how to respond to a newly thin mate.

If your surgery is affecting your marriage, you may want to consider marriage counseling along with any support groups you are participating in after your procedure.

You may find that as you lose weight, your self-esteem improves and your tolerance for bad behavior from your significant other is decreased. In the past you may have felt no one else would be interested in you, but feeling attractive makes you realize that there are others with whom you could have a relationship.

Substance Abuse When Food Is No Longer a Drug

If you have been using food as a drug, eating to help you cope with emotions and feelings you may not want to deal with, you may find yourself drawn to other addictive behaviors after surgery. Your stomach may not be able to accommodate much food, but it can, unfortunately, accommodate alcohol, and many drugs bypass the stomach altogether.

If you don't deal with the emotions and problems that drove you to overeat before surgery, you might be at greater risk for turning to other substances and behaviors after surgery. Getting to the root of those issues and developing coping mechanisms may help prevent moving from a food addiction to another form of addiction.

Why should I be worried about addiction issues when I'm conquering my food addictions so easily?
People who have an addictive personality—that is, people who are predisposed to addictive behaviors—can switch addictions when they are no longer able to get their "drug." In the case of weight loss surgery, it may no longer be possible to use food as a drug, so in times of stress, drugs and alcohol may be a tempting way to numb feelings.

Drugs and Alcohol

Drugs and alcohol, like food, can be used to avoid dealing with unwanted feelings and emotions. Some people will stop using food to control what they are feeling and can successfully lose weight that way, but they use drugs or alcohol in place of food. In terms of health and well-being, drugs and alcohol can be just as bad, if not worse, than an addiction to food.

Sex

Many people say that they feel sexually liberated after having lost significant amounts of weight. They are more comfortable in their own skin, and are far more interested in having sex. In most cases, these are very positive things, allowing people to enjoy their lives more fully. However, in some cases, sex can act as a replacement for a food addiction, much like drugs and alcohol.

A healthy sex life is not a problem, but an unhealthy sex life can be a major issue. If you are behaving recklessly and seeking out partners to fulfill an emptiness inside that food used to fill, you may want to consider seeking therapy. Sex addiction exists, and it is more likely to happen in people who have other types of addictions in their past, such as a food addiction.

CHAPTER 7

Exercise after Weight Loss Surgery

Without exercise, your weight loss plans are unlikely to be as successful as you hope. Eating right is only half the battle. Without exercise, your weight loss will be slower, you'll be less likely to reach your goal weight, and it will be more difficult to maintain your weight. The good news is that you do not have to be out running marathons on weekends to reap the benefits of exercise.

The Benefits of Exercise

You've heard it before; exercise is good for your health. What you may not have heard is that it is incredibly important to you, as a weight loss surgery patient, to start an exercise program and stick with it. The benefits of surgery—including weight loss, reversing health conditions, and improved levels of energy—are all heightened by exercise.

After your surgery you will lose weight rapidly, especially in the first six months after your procedure. During those months exercise will help you maintain muscle mass; burn more calories; and in some cases, help prevent the overabundance of skin that many people face after tremendous weight loss. In the long term, exercise will help you continue to lose and maintain that loss. Exercise can help you "make up" for eating too many calories, and can allow you to eat more calories without gaining weight.

The physical benefits are not limited to better health and weight loss. Exercise can improve the way you look and feel. You'll have far more energy when you include exercise in your day-to-day life, and your physical appearance will improve as well. Firm and well-toned muscle will improve the way your entire body looks. It will help your skin "shrink" to fit your smaller body and will make your body more defined.

Lower Blood Pressure

Exercise has been proven to lower blood pressure. Combined with significant weight loss and a healthy diet, many people who have high blood pressure are able to maintain a normal blood pressure without medication. Exercise may allow you to say goodbye to the side effects of blood pressure medication forever.

ALERT

If you are on blood pressure medication, be sure to have your blood pressure checked regularly after your surgery. Your blood pressure may return to normal as you lose weight and exercise, which, combined with medication, can actually make your blood pressure too low. Check with your doctor before making any changes to your blood pressure medication.

Lower Cholesterol

Your cholesterol levels can be expected to decrease as your exercise program and weight loss get into high gear. The combination of a low fat diet and exercise is an especially potent combination in the battle against cholesterol. Not only can you expect your bad (LDL) cholesterol to decrease, but you may also see a beneficial increase in your good cholesterol (HDL). In fact, research has shown that exercising four or more times per week can significantly boost your levels of good cholesterol (HDL). Even a moderate increase in your HDL can help protect you from heart disease.

Increased Weight Loss

Exercise helps improve weight loss in more than one way. Every calorie that you burn, as long as you have not eaten too many calories that day, can contribute to your weight loss. If you walk for an hour, you may burn as many as 400–500 calories, depending on your current weight, how hard your body is working during that time, and other factors.

That isn't the only positive aspect of exercise. You don't just burn calories while you are exercising, your metabolic rate can be increased for hours after you arrive home from the gym, providing many hours of enhanced calorie burning. Exercise will also increase your lean muscle mass, which will increase the number of calories that you burn on a daily basis. Your metabolism will increase as you continue to exercise, because your new muscle increases the number of calories your body requires to get through the day.

Control Type 2 Diabetes

Exercise can greatly improve type 2 diabetes, and in some cases, combined with dietary changes, can actually "cure" the condition. Many people who start exercising and begin losing weight find that they no longer need medication to control their blood glucose levels. In fact, successful weight loss patients often find that they have no signs or symptoms of diabetes as long as they meet and maintain their goal weight, or a healthy body weight.

Improved Skin Tone

If you are concerned about having excess skin after you reach your goal weight, you have an added incentive to start exercising. Aerobic exercise, such as walking, aerobics classes, bicycling, or other activities that increase your heart rate, can help minimize the excess skin you have in the long term.

Now, you aren't going to see your skin visibly shrink after your workout, but it will certainly help. Exercise can help your skin better conform to your new body, and will improve its appearance by toning muscles that lie under the skin. Combined with a diet rich in protein, good hydration, and a diet full of vitamins and nutrients, your skin could benefit greatly from your efforts.

Reduced Stress

Exercise is one of the best ways to relieve stress. Think of it as a two-for-one special: You reduce your stress and you speed your way to your goal weight. Exercise reduces stress in several ways. It stimulates the release of endorphins in your brain, leading to an enhanced feeling of well-being. This effect is often referred to as "runner's high."

Exercise is also known to improve mood. Having a bad day? Exercise may be just the thing you need. In addition, it makes an excellent substitute for some of the less-than-positive coping mechanisms you may have developed over the years. If you've had a bad day and you find that you have an almost irresistible urge to eat junk food, or binge, taking a walk or heading to the gym may be the ideal solution. Not only are you removing yourself from temptation, you are doing something good for your body and getting an emotional pick-me-up at the same time.

Improved Eating Habits

Can exercise really improve your eating habits? Yes and no. Yes, because many people who exercise regularly find that they are less likely to indulge or go off of their diet plan when they workout. They feel that going off of their diet plan would mean their workout was a waste of time, so they are more likely to adhere to their established diet guidelines.

Exercise can, however, increase appetite. It is important that you maintain hydration during your workout, and rehydrate after your workout. This will prevent you from overeating after a workout, when you are simply thirsty. If you have the urge to overeat after a workout, try having a low-calorie snack or starting your meal with a cup of broth-based soup, a small green salad, or fresh vegetables.

ALERT

> Many adults cannot tell the difference between hunger and thirst, and will eat when they are actually thirsty. Maintaining adequate hydration can prevent this, but if you are in doubt, drink a large glass of water and wait thirty minutes before eating.

Exercising Safely after Surgery

You will be encouraged to start exercising immediately after your surgery. Keep in mind that exercise means something very different the day after surgery than it does six months or a year after your procedure. Your ability to exercise will greatly increase as you get your strength back, and your stamina will increase as each pound comes off.

While it is a great idea to start exercising and start your exercise regime as quickly as possible, you will not be able to hop on a treadmill immediately after surgery. You can expect your stamina to be decreased after surgery, and pain will also limit how much you are able to accomplish initially.

The Days after Surgery

Exercise for someone recovering from surgery is very straightforward. The first day after surgery you will be expected to get out of bed and walk a few steps to a chair or the restroom. If you are able to tolerate sitting up in a chair and walking to the bathroom with minimal assistance, you will then start walking several times a day. Your walks may be brief, or you may be able to walk up and down the hallways. Staff will assist you during these short walks, making sure you are steady on your feet and preventing you from falling.

These short walks serve multiple purposes, helping to prevent blood clots and other surgical complications, in addition to getting you up on your feet as soon as possible. You should continue with these walks, and increase the length or duration of your walks, in the days and weeks following surgery. Your surgeon will tell you when you are cleared to begin a complete exercise program.

Exercise in the First Few Weeks

In the weeks immediately following your surgery, pain will be the major limiting factor of how much exercise you can do. It will be important to find a balance between not exercising enough and exercising too much, and causing more pain. Increasing exercise by a small amount each day is ideal. While you may only be able to make short walks initially, plan on adding more short walks or making each walk longer, as pain permits.

Low-impact exercise, such as walking, is ideal. While swimming is a fantastic low-impact exercise, plan on staying out of the pool until your incisions are completely closed. Once your incisions are healed, swimming, water walking, and water aerobics are great ways to get your heart pumping without putting additional stress on your joints.

After your procedure, your goal will be to manage your pain so that you are able to breathe normally, taking deep breaths, and you are able to walk short distances. If you are unable to control your pain well enough to do these things, it is important that you contact your surgeon. During a normal recovery, you should notice the pain start to slowly subside on a daily basis after the first few days. If you experience a sudden increase in pain, while walking or otherwise, it is important to be aware that this could be a sign of a complication.

Your surgeon will let you know when you are considered fully recovered from surgery and able to do whatever physical activities you desire. Until you are officially cleared for exercise, refrain from lifting heavy weights of any kind and any exercise that exclusively uses the abdominal muscles, such as crunches.

Stretching and More

Gentle stretching is an excellent way to ease soreness after surgery and increase flexibility. As with all exercise after surgery, your level of pain should be your guide, indicating when you may be pushing too hard too soon. While a full yoga routine will be too strenuous immediately after your procedure, slow and steady stretching, such as standing and bending at the waist to the sides and back, can be beneficial. You should avoid stretches that pull on the surgical incisions, or cause pain directly in the incision.

Once You Are Cleared for Exercise

Once your surgeon clears you for exercise, you will be able to participate in whatever physical activities you desire. This is great news, meaning you are no longer limited in your activities, but proceed with caution. What feels good on Monday may feel awful on Tuesday if you overdo your workout.

Start slowly with your first few workouts until you determine how your body will react to your new activity. If you were working out prior to your surgery, don't assume that you can leap back into the same workout. Your body has undergone a fairly radical change, as well as a few weeks away from the gym, so plan on having to gradually work back up to your prior workouts.

Getting Started

Getting started with a workout plan can be a daunting task, especially if it has been months, or even years, since you last exercised. It is important to keep in mind that exercise, especially if you are just getting started, is just activity that gets your heart beating faster. Exercise can be fifteen minutes of dancing around the house, walking around the neighborhood, or even raking leaves.

You can start as simply as walking for fifteen or twenty minutes, or even less if you are unable to exercise for extended periods of time. The goal is to get moving and increase how much you move over time. Regardless of your starting point, slowly increasing your workouts until you can exercise longer and harder is the goal.

Don't be intimidated by exercise. There are classes, exercise videos, and even online workout programs that are designed for people who are beginners, intermediate, and advanced.

Exercise If You Can't Walk

If you have difficulty walking, or bearing weight for any length of time, don't give up on exercise. There are multiple ways that you will be able to get your heart rate up without hurting yourself. You can modify workout tapes by doing the arm portion of the workout while sitting in a chair. As you get better and improve your stamina, you can do the same workout with weights to increase the intensity of the workout.

Isometric exercises, such as resistance bands, yoga, and Pilates, can often be done without bearing weight or standing. These exercises will strengthen your muscles and are great for toning.

Water exercise is also a great way to do a workout without bearing weight. Water walking, water aerobics, and swimming are all nonimpact activities, but can provide an excellent aerobic workout. You can burn as many calories in the water as you can on land, but the activity is less strenuous for those who cannot tolerate walking and standing.

Personal Trainer

A personal trainer is a great way to get into an effective exercise program to burn fat and lose inches. A personal trainer can create an exercise plan just for you, focused on meeting your individual goals. You will be able to create a set of workouts, both aerobic and anaerobic, designed to increase the rate at which you burn calories and to improve your muscle tone.

There are benefits and disadvantages to hiring a personal trainer. While the guidance and planning that a personal trainer can provide is invaluable, a personal trainer can be very expensive. Keep in mind that you don't have to have a personal trainer present for every workout you do. A trainer can design a workout for you that you are able to follow independently. You can check back in periodically for adjustments to your workout. You can also sign up for a group session with a personal trainer, where you and a workout buddy can share the trainer's time for an hour at a time, which will significantly decrease the cost.

Exercise Classes

Exercise classes come in a variety of forms, ranging from beginner stretching classes to high-impact, high-energy classes that are very challenging. These classes typically are very motivational, with an instructor and music, which many find encouraging. You may also experience a positive kind of "peer pressure" where you feel challenged to complete the class because of the people around you.

There are classes that focus on muscle toning and building, classes that focus on stretching and flexibility, and classes that are meant to make you break a sweat and burn calories. You may find one class that you do religiously, or you may prefer to participate in a wide variety of classes to keep things interesting.

Aerobic Exercise

The word "aerobic" means "with oxygen" and aerobic exercise is activity that gets the heart beating faster and lungs breathing harder. Most exercise is aerobic, including walking, biking, running, exercise classes, swimming, and more.

Aerobics are the best type of exercise for fat burning and conditioning. Over time, with regular workouts that slowly increase in intensity, you will be able to work out harder and longer, burning more calories with each workout. As your stamina improves, you will find that you have to make your exercise harder to get the same level of workout. For example, when you first start exercising, it may be difficult to walk a mile, but after a few months, you may find that walking a mile is no longer a challenge and you need to add a longer distance or walk much faster to increase your heart rate.

Common Types of Aerobic Exercise

The most common types of aerobic exercise are walking, swimming, and biking. All of these activities take a variety of forms; for example, you can take a stroll for your walk, or you can race walk, which is walking at a pace like a jog. Swimming may mean hopping into the pool and swimming laps, but water aerobics are also a great way to experience a low impact workout in water. You may enjoy biking around your neighborhood, or you can sign up for a high energy spinning class, which is an aerobic workout that is tough to beat in terms of the number of calories burned.

If you have a favorite aerobic workout, be sure to look for variations on that theme. It will help keep you interested in exercise and may improve your weight loss efforts.

Anaerobic Exercise

Anaerobic exercise includes activities that build or tone muscle or that require short bursts of exertion. While the term "anaerobic" is most often used with bodybuilding and weight training, it also includes quick bursts of running, biking, or other activities that might otherwise be thought of as aerobic.

While anaerobic workouts may not burn as many calories as aerobic workouts, they do increase fat burning long term by building muscle tissue, which increases metabolism. Balancing your workouts between anaerobic and aerobic exercise will help increase your overall fat burning and weight loss.

How Much, How Often?

The amount of exercise you can do today, and your exercise goals may be very different. You should aim for an hour of exercise no less than five times per week to maximize your weight loss and your ability to maintain your weight. Initially, especially in the first few weeks after your procedure, that goal will probably not be realistic. You should see how much activity you are safely able to accomplish, then slowly add more time and intensity to your workouts.

ESSENTIAL

Plan on working out every other day at the least. An excellent rule of thumb is this: If you didn't work out yesterday, you have to work out today. This will mean you work out at least three times a week one week, followed by four workouts the next week.

How Hard Should You Be Working Out?

The primary goal of your workouts at this point will be fat burning, so it is important that you work out at the right intensity to meet that goal. Your target heart rate will help you determine if you are working out hard enough (or too hard) for fat burning. First, subtract your age from 220. Then multiply that number by .65, which will give you the low end of your target range. Then multiply that number by .85, which is the high end of your target heart rate.

For example, if you are forty years old:

$220 - 40 = 180$

$180 \times .65 = 117$

$180 \times .85 = 153$

This means the target range for someone forty years of age is 117 to 153 heartbeats per minute.

So what does the target heart range tell you? In this example, you should be exercising hard enough that your heart beats at least 117 times per minute, but not so hard that it is beating faster than 153 times per minute. Working out too hard will limit your fat burning; not working out hard enough won't burn fat, and you won't improve your cardiovascular fitness.

Taking your pulse (heart rate) is not difficult. Using your index finger and middle finger, feel for a pulse on your neck, below your jaw and alongside your windpipe. Be sure to press gently, or you may not be able to feel your pulse. You can also feel your pulse on your wrist, near your thumb. It will be easier to feel a pulse when you are working out, since your heart will be beating harder and faster than it does when you are at rest.

FACT

While you are working out, you won't want to stop for an entire minute and take your pulse. Instead, take your pulse for ten seconds, and then multiply the number of heart beats by six. This will tell you how many times your heart is beating in one minute.

New Activities

Adding new activities to your workout can help you lose weight, but it can also help you enjoy your workouts more. It is easy to become bored with a treadmill, spending hours in the same place, and the same is true of many types of exercise. Don't be afraid to try new activities that aren't currently part of your plan. Team sports, such as soccer or volleyball, offer an amazing workout and can add fun to it.

While many nontraditional activities can be fun and also burn calories, they may not be as effective as your traditional workout. Consider joining an adult recreational league, which will help by putting team events on your calendar, and introduce you to other people interested in athletics.

You may find household activities that are not typically considered exercise, but certainly provide activity and calorie burning, such as mowing, gardening, or chopping wood. While these won't replace your trips to the gym, they certainly help burn calories.

You may also find ways to make your current workout more difficult, such as adding hand weights to your walks, or walking in the sand on a beach instead of on a road. You may want to ask friends to join in while you exercise, which can help make the time pass more quickly and certainly can make working out more fun.

Increasing Your Activity

You will want to increase your exercise at a moderate pace, so that you don't hurt yourself or overdo it. Once you are fully recovered from your surgery, you will have a better idea of how hard and how long you are able to work out without being exhausted and feeling as though you are ready to collapse. Consider this workout your baseline, the exercise you are able to accomplish without injuring yourself, or doing too much too fast.

Once you know your baseline, you can start building toward your goal of working out for an hour. Be realistic in your goal: If you are currently walking for fifteen minutes, your goal for next month should not be to run for an hour. Plan on adding 10 percent to your workout each week, until you are able to exercise for a full hour. This means if you are currently walking twenty minutes, next week you should walk twenty-two minutes. The week following, you will add another 10 percent, which would be twenty-four or twenty-five minutes.

If you are able to progress more quickly than 10 percent per week, that is great! You may find that as you shed pounds you are able to exercise harder and longer than you thought possible without feeling exhausted.

Measuring Success

While it is tempting to rely on the scale to determine how successful your efforts have been, exercise gives you more ways to measure your success. Tracking your progress of how long you are able to exercise and at what intensity should clearly show your accomplishments. You will find that as you exercise for weeks or even months, you will be working out harder and longer, but it will be easier than it was initially. Getting fit is something to celebrate and it plays a major role in your long-term success, so these accomplishments should be noted.

The old saying about muscle weighing more than fat? It is absolutely true! On weeks when you are not satisfied with what the scale is saying, take your measurements. You may find that you've lost inches, but the scale hasn't budged. Moving into a smaller size, no matter what the scale says, is a sign of success and is just as important as pounds lost.

No Pain, No Gain

While the phrase "no pain, no gain," is common when you are discussing working out, the reality is that your workout should not cause you anything more than discomfort. A tough workout may leave you feeling breathless, or with a muscle cramp, or a "stitch" in your side. These things pass as you recover from exercise, catching your breath and cooling down. True pain, such as an injury, does not need to be part of your exercise plan.

If it causes pain, don't do it. You may be pushing too hard after your surgery and you may be doing harm to your body. Pain is your best guide to when you are overdoing, pushing too hard, or doing an unsafe activity. As you start to work harder during your exercise session, you will learn to differentiate the normal discomfort after a hard workout from true pain.

CHAPTER 8

Wardrobe Issues

One of the major challenges you will face while on your weight loss journey is maintaining an adequate wardrobe while your clothing size is constantly changing. Being able to buy smaller sizes should be fun, as long as you don't let the expense cause too much stress.

Assessing Your Closet

Taking a long, hard look at your closet will help you in multiple ways. If you don't take the time to clean out all of the clothes that are no longer appropriate for you, you won't be able to tell at a glance if you have enough clothing to get you through the week. Your clothing size will be changing fairly rapidly, especially in the first six months after your surgery, so having a closet that works for you is a great idea.

It is time to expose your wardrobe, including your closet, dresser drawers, underbed storage, and armoire to the light of day. Do you have clothes in the attic that you haven't looked at for years? Do you have a laundry pile that you never get to the bottom of, and have no idea what lurks deep within? It is time to take an honest look at your clothes; decide what you like and what you won't wear; and even more importantly, get an inventory of what will work for you in the coming months.

Assessing what you have and how it suits your needs and future needs will help tremendously for the next step: cleaning out your closet. If you are doing this prior to surgery and you have some loose pants, and things that are less likely to rub against your incisions, set those aside for your recovery period. Ideally, they will have an elastic waist band or a drawstring waist, so you can tweak the fit.

Cleaning Out Your Closet

It's time to start weeding through your wardrobe from top to bottom. All of your clothing, from undergarments and pajamas to casual wear to formal wear, needs to be sorted through so you can decide if it should stay or go. In many cases, this should be very easy, but it is also easy to form an emotional attachment to your favorite pieces of clothing, so don't feel that you have to be utterly ruthless in purging your closet, unless you need the space.

Clothing That Is Too Large

The easiest way to start cleaning out is with clothing that is too big today. As you will be losing a significant amount of weight, there is no reason to hold on to any clothing that is too large. Even if it is only moderately large now, within weeks of your surgery it will not be wearable and should go into your discard pile.

Clothing That Is Outdated

Another category of clothing that can be easily purged from your wardrobe is anything that is outdated. Of course, if you have an outfit that is special to you, regardless of size or your ability to wear it, such as a wedding dress or something that you wore on a special occasion, by all means keep it. However, if it is obviously last year's style, or even older than that, you'll probably want to put it in the discard pile.

Clothing That Is Damaged or Needs Alterations

Do you have a pair of pants that needs to be hemmed, or a shirt with a button that needs to be sewn on? Consider getting rid of it. If you haven't gotten around to fixing it already, what is the likelihood that you will do so before it no longer fits? Do you want to invest your time or energy into fixing the clothing just to find that you can't wear it anyway? Favorite pieces might be an exception, but the vast majority of apparel that isn't wearable today will never be worn again, so the best place for it is probably in the discard pile.

Clothing That Is Worn Out

If your jeans have holes in them, or your underwear is no longer white no matter how much bleach you use, they should probably hit the discard pile, regardless of their size. You want to enjoy the clothes you are wearing on your shrinking body, not wear clothing that isn't as nice as it could be. If you don't get rid of them now, you may be tempted to wear those ratty jeans instead of getting a new pair that looks nice and fits properly. It is expensive to replace clothing, but you want to celebrate your new size, not feel trapped in clothing that you don't like just because it is the right size.

Clothing You Never Wore

It's the right size. It fits nicely. So what's the problem? You never wore it in the first place! Something about it just didn't suit you, so maybe you wore it once, or you never even took it off the hanger. Maybe you meant to return it, but never got around to it, so it sits in your closet. Or perhaps it was a well-meaning gift that wasn't quite right.

The reality is this: If you don't like it, have no desire to wear it, and really don't care if it fits or not, into the discard pile it goes!

Wrong Season

If you have clothing that fits, but it is a pair of shorts and it is the middle of January, you will probably want to place it in the discard pile. By the time the season rolls around, you will be several sizes smaller and the clothing will no longer fit, so don't feel that you have to wait until it is the right season to get rid of it.

There may be some items that you aren't sure you want to part with. For example, you may be able to squeak more wear out of a winter coat with a belt, but you know you'll never be tempted to wear the XXXL sweatshirt that lurks at the back of your closet. It's okay to keep the first and toss the latter.

You Don't Like It or Want It

Much like clothing that you never wore in the first place, don't keep things that you don't like, regardless of the size. If a piece of clothing is not appealing to you, it won't matter if the fit is beautiful or if the color makes your eyes look wonderful, you simply won't wear it. The clothing you keep should make you happy, or at the very least it should make you think, "I'd like to wear that a few more times before it doesn't fit."

There may also be clothing that you no longer want, such as dress clothes when you no longer have a job that requires a dressier wardrobe. If you don't want it, toss it. There is no need to feel guilty about it, the new you deserves clothes that are appealing.

What to Do with Clothes You No Longer Need or Want

Once you've gone through your wardrobe, sorting out the things you want to keep, you will probably have a large quantity of clothes that you need to find a new home for. Don't worry, those clothes can do a lot of good for you and for others, and they don't need to be thrown away unless they are absolutely unwearable.

The best thing to do is to sort the clothes that you will not be keeping into three piles or boxes; one for charitable donation, one to share, and one to sell if there is a resale shop in your area.

Sharing Your Old Clothing

If you are taking part in a support group for bariatric patients, consider sharing your old clothing with your fellow support-group patients. You will all be experiencing the same rapid change in weight and size, so you may be able to save each other a tremendous amount of money by sharing clothing. Many support groups establish a monthly clothing swap. Each person brings their gently used clothing that no longer fits, then tables of clothes are set up by size. You bring the clothing that you no longer want, and go home with new clothing that you can enjoy until it no longer fits, then repeat the process.

Even some weight loss surgery groups that meet online do clothing swaps, as the cost of postage is the only cost for trading. It is helpful to swap with someone who has similar clothing needs as you, such as someone who works in a professional environment and must wear dress clothes, or someone who has many casual clothes such as jeans.

Selling Clothing

If the clothes you are discarding are mostly professional apparel or are in excellent condition, you may want to consider selling them via a resale shop. Not only will you be paid for your unwanted clothing, but many shops will give a greater amount of in-house credit than they will give cash. As you will be needing clothes in a variety of sizes, credit at a resale shop may be beneficial.

Resale shops require clothing to be clean, neatly folded or ironed, and free of any stains or defects. They are also willing to accept shoes, in most cases, provided that they are not overly worn.

Donating Clothing

If you have a local charity that accepts clothing donations, donating your clothing is not only an act of kindness, you will be entitled to use the donation as a deduction on your income taxes. You will have to obtain a receipt for your donation, so dropping off a bag at a collection drop site won't be possible, but in exchange for your efforts, you can save money.

A good rule of thumb for the deduction is 25 percent of the original purchase price of the garment, but you will want to speak to your tax preparer regarding the deduction to be sure.

ALERT

Save all of your clothing receipts if you are planning to make any donations to a charity that accepts clothing. This will make it easier to defend your tax deduction if any questions should arise from the IRS when you file your taxes.

Organizing Your Newly Clean Closet

Now that you've gotten rid of all of the clothes that you no longer want or need, it is time to make your closet accessible and make it work for you. How you organize your closet is really up to you, but if the clothes you kept cover a wide range of sizes, you may want to organize by size, rather than by type of clothing or by color. This way, as you move into a smaller size, you can see at a glance what needs to be removed from your closet. It's a long-held belief that when you are on a serious weight loss plan you should get rid of clothes that are too big, the idea being that if you don't have any clothes that are larger you will be more motivated to maintain your weight loss.

Organizing by size will also help you keep up on your closet organization. You won't have to repeat the entire process to remove clothing that doesn't fit; you can just remove all the clothes in the section designated for the clothes of that size.

Buying Clothing

As you lose weight, buying new clothing is unavoidable. Your body will be changing so much, and often so rapidly, that you may find yourself shopping more than you ever have in the past. While it may be irritating at times to make a purchase only to find that it no longer fits six weeks later, try to take joy in the process of shedding pounds and needing smaller clothes.

Buy Minimally

When you start buying clothing for your new body, you may be tempted to buy a considerable amount of clothing. It might be wiser to stick with the basic essentials, as you may be in and out of a size in only a few weeks, so your investment will pay only short-term rewards.

A few pairs of pants or skirts along with some shirts may be able to get you through the work week, and a pair of jeans or casual pants might be enough for the weekend. You are the best judge of your needs in terms of how much clothing you need for your day-to-day life, but buying less clothing in each size may help ease the transition. This is especially true in the first six months, when your weight loss will be the most rapid and may result in changing sizes once a month or even more frequently.

Basics

Basic wardrobe essentials are different for everyone. A dress shirt, suit, and tie may be one person's work basic, while khakis and a polo shirt might be work wear for someone else. In any case, sticking with your basics will help ease the transition through sizes without breaking the bank.

For example, if you have to wear a suit to work, you would be far better served with a basic gray suit than you would with a suit that is a notable color or only goes with one tie. The gray suit can be paired with a variety of ties and shirts, making it look like an entire new outfit, without the expense of purchasing multiple suits. Dress shirts are far less expensive to replace than an entire suit.

In a business casual office, a pair of khaki pants may be your staple, and purchasing a few shirts that match may be all you need to do to be appropriately attired. For casual wear, many people consider jeans a must-have, so they too would be considered a basic wardrobe piece.

Mix and Match

If you are changing sizes rapidly, or prefer not to spend a tremendous amount of money on clothes that will only fit for a few weeks or months, consider purchasing only items that match. For example, if you purchase a pair of khaki pants and a pair of navy pants and three shirts that match both pairs of pants, you've essentially created six outfits. This type of strategic purchasing can help stretch your wardrobe dollars and greatly increase your options when deciding what to wear each day.

You know your wardrobe needs, but planning to have everything interchangeable can really help maximize your clothing while minimizing your expenses.

Adjustable Waists

Adjustable waistbands are your friend. If you are able to adjust the waist on your pants, whether it be with a drawstring or button tabs, you will be able to get a much longer life from them. The same is true of shirts. If you have a shirt or dress with a wrap waist, the fit can be altered as you change sizes, extending the wear considerably.

ESSENTIAL

When you are shopping for clothing it is important that you purchase items that either fit or are a bit on the snug side. This doesn't mean that you should purchase something that requires you to skip meals or breath shallowly in order to wear it, but your new clothes shouldn't be loose. Clothing that is on the larger side won't be wearable for nearly as long as something that was a proper fit when the purchase was made.

New Shoes

You may go into your weight loss journey thinking that your shoes won't need to be replaced. In many cases, that is not true. While the feet tend to change less than the rest of your body, they will change shape. Most importantly, the way your shoes fit will change as you continue to drop pounds. You may be able to tighten your laces to make shoes fit better, but some will just not fit well enough for you to continue wearing them.

As you replace your shoes, you may want to make a point of buying shoes that lace up, just because they are more adjustable. If that is not possible, keep an eye on the fit and how your feet feel. If you start to feel like you are walking out of your shoes, or if they don't offer the support or comfort that they have in the past, it may be time to replace them.

You may find that slip-on shoes, with no laces or fasteners, are not an ideal option as you lose weight, because they become too loose as you lose weight. If you find that your slip-ons no longer want to stay on, you should probably replace them. You may want to skip slip-on shoes altogether until your weight stabilizes or you are close to your goal weight.

FACT

As you lose weight, you may want to have your feet measured by a shoe store staff member. Your feet may actually change sizes, or they may become more narrow as you lose weight. The better your shoes fit, the better your feet will feel, so don't hesitate to make sure your shoe size hasn't changed before you make a purchase.

Workout Shoes

Your workout shoes are a bit different than your day-to-day shoes. If you are working out religiously, three or more times a week, your shoes will no longer provide adequate support once you've been wearing them three to six months. If your workout shoes no longer feel supportive, don't fit as well as they once did, or feel like they don't offer the protection from the impact that you feel during exercise, it is time to shop for a new pair.

Your feet will take a considerable pounding when you work out, especially if you are running, walking, or playing sports. A poorly fitted athletic shoe, or one that no longer provides support, can lead to foot pain and injury so replacing them regularly is very important.

Clothing You Shouldn't Buy

When you are losing weight, you will absolutely need to purchase new clothes, but you can minimize the amount of clothing you must purchase by buying with a few parameters in mind. If you are someone who wants to minimize the expense of replacing your wardrobe regularly, keeping a few guidelines in mind will help you considerably.

Future Seasons

Don't plan on buying clothing for future seasons unless you are approaching your goal weight, as it is very difficult to predict what size you will be wearing in several months. If you buy too far ahead, you may find that you can't wear the item when the appropriate season rolls around.

While the shorts that are on sale may seem like an ideal purchase, it is frustrating when it is sunny outside and the shorts are so large that they want to fall off, or you haven't quite gotten into that size yet. Making a purchase when you need it, rather than for a need you may have in the future, will prevent you from wasting money on clothing you never have an opportunity to wear, and allow you to purchase what you want when you want it.

Baggy or Oversized

If you are like many people, you don't often buy clothes that truly fit. You may buy clothes that are baggy, or even too big. You may buy clothing that is cut to be oversized, rather than more tailored in appearance. In order to truly maximize your wardrobe, you will want to buy clothing that fits on the day you purchase it, or is perhaps a tiny bit on the snug side.

Shirts tend to be more forgiving of weight loss, but pants especially should be purchased while they fit appropriately. The lifespan of a pair of pants during weight loss can be very short, as they have a tendency to fall down when they are significantly too large. At some point even a belt can't make pants fit properly, so avoid the purchase of baggy pants.

Clothing That You Don't Try On

It will be much easier for you to make purchases in a store, rather than online or from a catalog while you are losing weight rapidly. It is easy to inaccurately estimate your current size, and often your body shape will change so radically that cuts that would have fit beautifully and have been flattering in the past just don't work now. There are exceptions to every rule, and if you can finally fit into the cashmere sweater of your dreams, certainly don't let the lack of a changing room stop you. The vast majority of your purchases, however, shouldn't be made without trying things on or you may find yourself spending your time making returns at stores instead of shopping for new clothing.

FACT

> Your size may change rapidly, especially in the early months after surgery. Don't be surprised if something that fit when you bought it does not fit two weeks later. For this reason, it is best to allow extra time for trying on clothing when shopping, even when purchasing brands and clothing you are confident will fit.

Getting a Few More Weeks Out of Your Clothes

Getting a few extra weeks out of your clothing may allow you to save money, or even to skip buying a size altogether. If nothing else, if you don't enjoy shopping, you may be able to spend those few weeks without buying more clothes. In addition to buying clothes that fit, or are a bit snug, you can always wear your clothes a bit baggier than you might otherwise. Of course, this may mean that your weight loss isn't quite as noticeable and isn't an option for some who prefer a more tailored appearance.

Stretch fabrics can be both a blessing and a curse. Some allow for greater size flexibility and can be purchased in a smaller size than a traditional fabric, so they can be worn longer than traditional fabrics as your weight loss continues. Others tend to stretch too much, and end up being too large too soon. Pay attention to the label if you are buying stretch fabrics, it will tell you what percentage of the material is stretchy, such as spandex, and what portion is not going to stretch, such as cotton.

Belts and Suspenders

Belts will be your friends as you change sizes, and for men, suspenders are equally helpful. A good belt is the best way to get more wear from your pants and jeans. If you like using a belt to get more mileage out of your clothing, look for pants with belt loops rather than waistless styles and elastic waist bands.

Tailors

If you have a piece of clothing that you absolutely love but can no longer wear, tailoring may be just what you need. A good tailor can make your pants, suits, and shirts smaller, but it comes at a price. Tailors can often be more expensive than the cost of a replacement garment, but if you really enjoy wearing something, the fee they charge may be well worth it. As you approach your goal weight and you change sizes more slowly, tailoring may be a better option, as you won't be approaching a new size shortly after the alterations are complete.

If you are handy with a needle and thread, you may be able to do simple alterations yourself. Taking in a waistband or putting darts in a shirt will help you get much more wear out of your clothing, and will save you a significant amount of money as your size gets smaller and smaller.

Pin It and Cover It

So you have some pants that don't quite fit anymore, but you aren't interested in replacing them. You can put a belt on, but the waistband looks a bit funny because you've cinched it down so much. What's the solution? Cover the waistband. A jacket, sweater, or even a shirt that doesn't need to be tucked in can cover that bunched-up waist.

Some people swear by safety pins, using them to make a shirt smaller by pinning the back, then covering it with a jacket or sweater. Some people insist that a stash of safety pins is an absolute necessity for another reason: Some of the new fabrics used to make clothing stretch may work too well, and what fits during the morning may be trying to fall down in the afternoon.

CHAPTER 9

How to Eat and Drink after Weight Loss Surgery

Dietary changes are essential after having weight loss surgery. Having surgery isn't the answer, it is the first step to losing weight, and the way you eat after your procedure is what will determine how successful you are at weight loss. Weight loss surgery is not a cure-all: If your diet doesn't change, no surgery can provide the results you are looking for.

Dietary Restrictions after Weight Loss Surgery

After your surgery, your ability to eat will be radically changed. In the days following surgery, food may not be an option, with sips of water being the extent of what you are able to tolerate. Over the next weeks, and even months, you will slowly increase your food intake until you are able to tolerate meals that are nearly a cup in size.

The tiny size of meals will help kick-start your weight loss. You can expect, if you follow your doctor's instructions, to have significant weight loss in the initial weeks following your procedure.

The radical decrease in the amount of food you are able to eat during a meal is not the only change that you will be making. The foods you choose to eat should change considerably as well. The new staple of your diet will become lean protein, along with whole grains and fresh fruits and vegetables.

While you will be including new, lean foods in your diet, you will also need to eliminate foods that are diet killers. Fatty foods, empty calories, and junk foods will have to be banished from your day to day life if you want to have the best possible outcome from your surgery.

Clean Eating

Your new way of eating is referred to by a variety of names, most commonly as "clean eating" or "spa cuisine." These are just ways of describing food that is as fresh as possible, not processed, full of nutrients, and made with a minimum of additives. Proponents of clean eating often encourage the use of organic foods, raised without chemicals including chemical fertilizers, pesticides, and herbicides.

ALERT

One of the easiest things you can do to enhance your weight loss is to avoid drinking calories. It is very easy to consume far too many calories if they are in liquid form, such as soda or alcohol. Make an effort to eliminate liquid calories from your diet once you've moved past the liquid diet stage of your recovery.

Changing Tastes

The thought of eliminating fatty and sugary foods from your diet may seem scary, but it shouldn't. You will be amazed at how quickly your tastes change when you alter your diet. Within a few weeks of giving up fatty and salty foods, you will find that they don't taste the way you remember them.

French fries are a great example of foods that will taste differently when you stick with your diet and get used to the flavor and texture of foods that are lower in fat. After a few weeks or months of eliminating excess sodium and fat from your diet, you may be tempted by a treat like French fries. What might surprise you, however, is that they won't taste as good as you remember, but will taste greasy and salty. Use these changes in your tastes to your advantage. If the first bite doesn't taste good, don't take another.

The way your body reacts to food will also change. You may have been a chocolate addict before surgery but find that now even a nibble makes your stomach upset and triggers dumping syndrome or pain.

Lean foods, or foods low in fat, will comprise the vast majority of your diet. Keeping the fat content of your diet down will decrease the total number of calories you are taking in and will also promote positive health changes such as lower cholesterol.

What to Eat

If you are serious about weight loss, you need to be equally serious about what you eat. It isn't enough to limit the size of your meals, the food you choose is incredibly important. Regardless of the type of surgery you choose, it is essential that every calorie you consume is full of vitamins and nutrients.

When the size of your meals is strictly limited, each and every morsel needs to provide your body with what it needs. So while a candy bar may be small enough to be included in your diet, and may be low enough in calories to be accommodated by your meal plan, it will take the place of lean protein, and foods that are full of vitamins and fiber.

The right food choices will do more than help your weight loss, they will help you feel full of energy, build and maintain muscle mass, and keep you "regular." Immediately after your surgery, sticking with the right foods will help prevent stomach upset, pain, dumping syndrome, and other side effects.

Lean Protein

Protein will be the primary focus of your new diet. Meat, and other forms of protein, such as beans, will be necessary to help keep your energy level high and to minimize muscle mass loss as you lose weight. When you start exercising, protein will also help you add to your existing muscle mass.

Most bariatric surgeons recommend no less than sixty grams of protein per day once you are able to eat a full diet. In order to get that much protein into your diet, you may have to start each meal by eating the protein component first, then eating side dishes. That way you will have consumed the suggested amount of protein before getting too full with carbohydrates or whole grains.

While meat and fish are typically the first protein sources that come to mind, there are many vegetarian options available including: beans, tempeh, texturized vegetable protein (TVP), soy, tofu, seitan, and nuts (nuts can be high in fat, so eat in moderation).

ALERT

Many vegetarian protein alternatives are very healthy foods, but not all. Even if the food is vegetarian, you will still need to read the label carefully, looking for fat content and added sugar and to determine how many calories you will be consuming.

If you are having difficulty getting enough protein into your diet, you may want to consider protein powder. This powder can be added to foods such as smoothies and can increase your protein intake considerably without adding unnecessary fat and calories to your diet.

Dairy Foods

Dairy can be an excellent source of protein, but not all dairy foods are a good choice after weight loss surgery. For example, low-fat cheese is a good option, but ice cream, while a good source of protein, certainly isn't a diet food. Some weight loss patients are very sensitive to dairy foods and can become constipated or have an upset stomach after consuming cheese or milk. To prevent an upset stomach or other annoying issues, plan on starting with very small portions until you are sure that you won't have a negative reaction to these foods.

Many dairy foods are available in nonfat varieties, such as skim milk and nonfat cheese. Low-fat options are also available and may have better flavor and texture than the fat-free varieties. If you are used to full-fat dairy foods, such as whole milk, you may not enjoy the taste of the lower-fat variety. In this case, consider using skim milk when cooking, and minimize the amount of milk you drink.

Following are some sources of low-fat dairy protein:

- Cottage cheese
- Cheese
- Milk (preferably skim)
- Yogurt
- Frozen yogurt (low-fat, low-sugar varieties)
- Sour cream
- Buttermilk (low fat)

Whole Grains

Whole grains are a great food for a variety of reasons. Not only are they high in fiber and nutrients, but they also provide lean protein in addition to carbohydrates. Including whole grains in your diet will increase satiety, making you feel full longer.

ESSENTIAL

Whole grain is becoming more and more common in the foods available at the supermarket. Many cereals, breads, and even snacks are now available with whole grains rather than more refined flour. Be sure the label says "whole grain" as "whole wheat" is not the same thing.

Reading labels will be very important in making sure you get enough whole grains in your diet. Flour that is highly refined is white flour, and it is the least desirable type of flour for your diet, as it has less fiber and nutrients than whole wheat flour. Look for labels that say "whole grain" and choose these options rather than the ones that are made with refined flour. Breads, pastas, and rice, when eaten, should all be the less processed varieties, such as whole-grain brown rice, rather than instant white rice.

Some whole-grain sources include:

- Popcorn
- Oats (such as oatmeal)
- Barley (great in soup or as a hot cereal)
- Pasta
- Bread
- Brown rice
- Wild rice
- Whole-grain tortillas
- Buckwheat
- Bulgur
- Whole wheat flour
- Quinoa

QUESTION

What is the difference between whole grain and whole wheat?
"Whole grain" means that the grain is not processed and remains whole. Whole grain is difficult for the body to process, which adds fiber to your diet. "Whole wheat" has all the same nutrients, but is far more processed, and not as beneficial to your body. It is easier to digest, but your system doesn't get the benefit of the fiber.

Fruit and Vegetables

Fresh fruits and vegetables will be your best sources of vitamins and minerals, and they are low in calories. A cup of lettuce, for example, has approximately 10 calories, which contrasts sharply with unhealthy foods such as butter, which packs a whopping 1,600 calories per cup.

When you are hungry and concerned about overeating, fruits and vegetables can fill the void without causing you to consume too many calories.

Avoid dry fruits. They often have added sugar and are much higher in calories than a similar-size serving of fresh fruit.

To get the most benefit, plan on eating a variety of fruits and vegetables in a range of colors. Think of the colors as providing different vitamins and minerals, so eating selections across the spectrum will ensure that you are obtaining the nutrients you need.

After fresh produce, frozen fruits and vegetables are your best option. They are available year-round and won't go bad in your refrigerator. Canned produce should be your last choice, as the level of vitamins and minerals is lower and often considerable amounts of sugar or salt are added in the canning process.

Your preparation of fruits and vegetables will be important to maintaining your diet. A perfectly healthful vegetable can become a diet-ruining disaster with the wrong cooking techniques. For example, a baked potato is a great option if you top it with a butter spray or low-fat chili. It is filling and nutritious, high in fiber, and low in calories. Now, add butter, sour cream, cheese, and bacon bits and you have food that can easily account for half a day's calories or more. The same is true of food like broccoli; when topped with melted cheese it becomes a less attractive option.

Supplements

Even if you follow your diet to the letter, a supplement such as a daily multivitamin is important. A good multivitamin can help insure that you get enough calcium, along with other vitamins and minerals, and can help make up for any nutritional deficiencies you may have. If you had a gastric bypass procedure, your surgeon may recommend a prescription supplement that you will have to continue taking long after your weight loss is complete.

Quantity of Food and Drink

The quantity of food and liquid that you can tolerate will be radically different than what you were accustomed to prior to surgery. During the days following surgery, you may not be able to tolerate food at all, instead taking sips of water and adding additional liquids over time. Your first few meals will be pureed foods, blended into a smooth liquid. The portion will be tiny, one to two tablespoons in size.

Once you can tolerate pureed food, you will move on to soft foods, such as mashed potatoes or soup. Over a course of weeks, you will move from a soft diet to a full diet, meaning you can eat a typical diet with a wide range of foods and textures.

Once you are taking a full diet, you will slowly increase the amount of food that you eat during a meal. The process will continue over several months, but you should be eating your new "normal" meal size by six months. For most patients, this means approximately one cup of food per meal.

There is no benefit to rushing the process, and trying to take larger meals than your body is comfortable accommodating. Stretching your pouch should happen naturally, and forcing your body to take a larger meal than it should can cause an upset stomach, vomiting, and other uncomfortable side effects.

Snacking

Snacking should be avoided as much as possible, for reasons that go beyond calorie control. Studies show that patients who snack have notably less weight loss than their nonsnacking counterparts. Your focus should be on three balanced meals a day, with no snacks unless absolutely necessary. That doesn't mean you should go hungry and starve between meals, but it does mean that snacks should be the exception, not the rule.

Some healthy snacks include:

- Fat-free pudding
- Yogurt
- Fresh fruits
- Nuts

- Low-fat cheese
- Whole-grain crackers
- Raw vegetables
- Protein bar

When you eliminate snacking, you will be able to more easily identify when you are eating for emotional reasons rather than physical hunger. If you plan on snacking, you won't be listening for the physical cues that tell you when it is time to eat, and learning to listen to your body is one of the essential skills that you will need to learn.

A major part of the process of adapting successfully to life after weight loss surgery is eliminating eating that isn't necessary, which is eating that is not based on physical hunger. If you choose to snack on a regular basis, you may eliminate opportunities to identify emotional eating patterns that you might not be aware of.

Avoiding Pain

Some pain may be unavoidable after surgery, but what and how much you eat can contribute to the pain you feel once you've fully recovered from surgery. Eating too much can cause discomfort that ranges from mildly irritating to very painful. Poor food choices, including soda, sugary foods, and foods that expand after eating, can also cause significant pain.

It is easy to eliminate sugary foods from your diet, but foods that are acceptable on your plan still have the potential to cause pain. Foods that expand after eating, such as toast or dried foods, can seem fine when you eat them, but cause stretching of your pouch as they absorb liquid from your stomach. Hard foods, such as crackers or carrots, can also cause pain or cause a feeling of being "stuck" in the esophagus.

Each time you try a new food, try to take small bits, chew thoroughly, and only take a small portion until you are certain that you can eat it without hurting later.

Fluid Intake

Drinking adequate fluids, primarily water, is important after surgery. After surgery you will be limited to sips of water, but over time you will increase your intake until you are drinking at least sixty four ounces of fluid a day. It will probably take a concerted effort to drink enough water initially, and you should actually drink more if you are exercising on a regular basis.

While you will be drinking a substantial amount of water each day, you should not drink any liquid in the half an hour immediately before or after any meal, including snacks. Drinking fluids with meals will make you feel full before you have finished your meal. Depending on the type of surgery you had, you can actually flush food out of your stomach prematurely, even though your procedure may be designed to hold food in your stomach longer, prolonging the feeling of fullness.

Caffeine acts as a mild diuretic, causing your body to make more urine and causing mild dehydration. If you are unable to give up your caffeinated beverages, plan on increasing your water intake to compensate for the diuretic effects of coffee and tea.

Alcohol

Alcohol should be eliminated or minimized after your surgery. Alcohol has no nutritional value, making it an "empty calorie" food. If you do choose to drink alcohol, do so in moderation. Your ability to drink liquids is greater than your ability to eat food, so you can easily drink far more calories than you might think. If you find yourself drinking more than you did in the past, keep in mind that a small percentage of patients "trade" addictions, switching from a food addiction to other types of addiction, including a substance addiction such as alcohol.

ALERT

One alcoholic beverage or full calorie beverage per day can add up to a whopping number of calories over the course of a year. If you drink 200 calories per day, in the course of a year that means you've consumed an extra 73,000 calories and may mean you lose up to twenty-one pounds less.

Foods to Avoid

Avoiding "bad" foods sounds easier than it truly is. You may think that you just need to stay away from fast food, soda, and junk food, but that isn't the case. You will need to read labels carefully, looking for hidden fat, sugar, and any ingredient that you know will upset your stomach.

Foods you should avoid include:

- Acidic foods (until your recovery is over, they can irritate your suture lines)
- Foods that expand
- Fatty food
- Sugar-laden food
- Junk foods
- Fried foods

You may discover food that doesn't agree with your system, and it might be foods that you thoroughly enjoyed prior to your procedure. You might find certain textures or certain categories of food, such as raw vegetables, are a problem.

Hidden Sugar

Sugar is a problem whether or not you experience dumping syndrome. Sugar is high in calories, but those calories are empty, totally lacking in nutritional value. Avoiding sugar will help keep your caloric intake under control.

If you experience dumping syndrome, it is even more important that you eliminate sugar from your diet. The nausea, lightheadedness, and other symptoms are worth avoiding, but sugar is hiding in many places that you might not expect. For example, on the surface, spaghetti sauce seems like an ideal diet food. It is typically low in calories, is vegetable based, and is generally a healthful selection. That said, many spaghetti sauces found in the grocery store are loaded with sugar, and cause dumping syndrome.

Candy can pack a lot of sugar and calories into a very small portion, so it should be excluded from the diet entirely, or eaten rarely at the very least.

Listen to Your Body

Listening to your body for symptoms of hunger may be one of the hardest things that you will do after your procedure, but the most essential. In addition to learning what to eat, you will slowly learn when to eat, rather than just eating when the mood strikes.

Ideally, you will learn to eat when you are hungry, rather than because it is time to eat, or because you are stressed, having a bad day, or bored. It is not uncommon to come to the realization that you have a strong emotional tie to food, especially when you are unable to eat after surgery.

Don't fall into the trap of thinking that just because you've had surgery that you will be satisfied with a few nibbles of food. That may be true in the days or weeks immediately after surgery, but long term you will need to eat normal but small meals. You've heard all of your life that you should eat breakfast, and that is especially true after surgery. Since you will be eliminating snacking from your diet, a meal that will get you through the morning without starving is important.

Waiting for hunger and waiting until you are starving are very different things. If you wait until you are ravenously hungry, you are far more likely to overeat, resulting in pain or discomfort along with consuming too many calories. On the other side of things, eating when you aren't hungry can also cause pain and discomfort, as your stomach will hold food much longer than it did in the past.

Avoiding Poor Food Choices

When you are eating at home, reading labels is the first line of defense against poor food choices. If you stick with the essential food choices of lean protein, fresh fruits and vegetables, whole grains, and low-fat dairy, you should be able to make most of your meals with a minimum of research. If you choose to eat prepared and processed foods, reading labels can make your grocery trips seem like they will never end.

Processed foods, as a general rule, should be your last choice for meals. Cooking from scratch, with minimal added fat and using fresh ingredients is ideal, but not always realistic. Sandwiches, salads, and other foods that don't require cooking can help fill the gap. When it isn't possible to prepare your meals yourself, frozen foods can make a good substitute, in the form of microwaveable or ready-to-eat meals. Meals that come in a box or a can should be your last choice, as they are typically very high in calories, additives, and fats.

In some ways, a stop at a fast food restaurant is preferable to many processed foods. With the addition of healthy and light options in most restaurants, you may be able to find a salad, soup, or sandwich that is a better choice than something from a vending machine.

FACT

If you are starving and need something to eat, a fast food restaurant may be just what you need. A single taco or a single plain hamburger will not ruin your day calorie-wise, as long as it doesn't come with French fries, a large sugary soda, or another calorie-rich side dish. Try to find something high in fiber, like a salad, or high in protein, like a hamburger. You can always take the bun off if you are worried about the calories.

If you work outside the home, consider stashing a healthy meal in the freezer at work, or even in your desk drawer. By preparing ahead for circumstances that don't accommodate your diet, you can avoid a situation where you have to choose between going hungry and eating something that is an unhealthy choice.

Preparing doesn't just mean stocking up on good foods. Don't hesitate to clear out your cupboards, removing all the foods that you know you won't be able to eat or shouldn't eat. Removing temptation may be very helpful while you are adjusting to your new lifestyle.

Eating in Restaurants

Eating in a restaurant isn't impossible, but it may take some effort and planning. Many restaurants have their menus posted online, giving you an opportunity to identify acceptable menu selections, or alternatively, rule out the restaurant as a place where you would like to dine.

Pay particular attention to appetizers, and even the children's menu, if necessary. Appetizers come in the smaller-sized portions that you require, but not all of them are prepared in a way that is a good option. Low-fat, high-protein options, such as a shrimp cocktail, could be a fantastic option, while a basket of onion rings would not fit the bill.

The appetizer option only works if there is a small menu item available that fits your dietary needs. Otherwise, plan on ordering a full-size meal, but leaving as much as 80 percent on your plate, depending on the portion size. You will find that it is a rare restaurant that serves a portion size that doesn't encourage overeating, whether one has had weight loss surgery or not.

If you are looking for an item to order in a restaurant, there are some key words that you should look for in menu descriptions to let you know what foods to avoid:

- Fried or deep-fried
- Sautéed
- Candied
- Cream sauce or cream-based
- Bernaise
- Hollandaise
- Alfredo
- Gravy
- Cheese sauce
- Custard

The intention of the list isn't to deprive you of a lovely evening out, but to help you avoid foods that are not only high in calories, but could cause serious stomach upset. Most surgeons would tell you that having a treat once in a while, like a meal in a restaurant, regardless of how the food is prepared, isn't a bad thing. If you dine in restaurants regularly, you will need to be stricter about your menu selections.

The Salad Trap

A salad seems like a natural solution when trying to make a diet-friendly selection at a restaurant, but that isn't always the case. A simple salad with a low-fat or no-fat dressing is a safe bet, but restaurant salads are not normally that kind of salad. In a restaurant you're more likely to get a salad that has four ounces or more of dressing, bacon pieces, cheese, croutons, dried fruit, crunchy noodles, and any other number of toppings that you don't need.

Instead of the toppings that make salad a diet loser, consider adding toppings that boost the protein content of your salad, such as shrimp, chicken, or lean beef. You can also add low-fat toppings such as garbanzo beans and low-fat cheese and top it off with your own salad dressing.

If you prefer to use the dressing provided by the restaurant, be sure to ask for it on the side. The average restaurant portion of dressing contains hundreds of calories, and averages half a cup of dressing. With the dressing on the side you can determine how much you want on your salad, or even better, dip your fork before each bite of salad, which gives the flavor of the dressing with minimal calories.

CHAPTER 10

Grocery Shopping after Weight Loss Surgery

Shopping for groceries can be a challenge after your surgery. Initially, you may struggle with what to buy and how much you will need, and wonder if you are making the right purchases. Learn how to shop for what you need and how to avoid those purchases you might want, but know you should avoid.

Assessing Your Pantry

Before you head off to the grocery store in search of tasty foods that won't ruin your weight loss plans, it is essential that you take a long, hard look at your pantry, refrigerator, freezer, and spice rack. The goal is to prepare your kitchen to provide you with nutritious food, and to remove temptation at the same time.

Your kitchen, if it is a typical one, probably has some healthy and nutritious foods, along with expired food, junk food, food that you don't even like, and food that you have no plans to eat, ever. You may have a family, and that throws even more food into the mix. You may have the typical childhood staples of hot dogs and macaroni and cheese, and maybe you have beer in your refrigerator.

The goal of assessing your food stores is not to get rid of every food that has ever given you pleasure so that you can suffer with your new diet plan. "Diet" in this context doesn't refer to something you do for a few weeks, it is a way of eating for your new lifestyle, a long-term commitment and change. Your diet, or the food you eat, should be largely healthy and "clean" food, so your pantry should be stocked to make that possible.

Start by assessing the contents of your freezer and refrigerator. How much of what you see is something you actually want to eat? How much of that would your surgeon want you to eat? What is expired or freezer burned? Do the same for your pantry, and any dry storage you may have.

Do You Have the Essentials?

Stocking the essentials doesn't necessarily mean a trip to the grocery store that fills a cart and breaks the bank. Essentials are the vital basics, along with some extras that help perk up flavor and make a meal complete. These foods should make up the vast majority of your diet, and will greatly contribute to your success if you eat them with portion control in mind.

ESSENTIALS INCLUDE:

- A variety of fresh vegetables (frozen if necessary)
- A variety of fresh fruits (frozen if necessary)

- Protein, such as fish, beef, pork, chicken, seafood, fish, or vegetarian meat substitutes
- Whole-grain bread, pasta, or cereal
- Low-fat or fat-free dairy
- Herbs and spices

In the days immediately after your surgery, the portions you will be eating will be petite, so the quantities you will require of each food group will be very small. Ideally, your surgeon will provide you with proper portion sizes for each stage of your recovery and weight loss plan, so you can easily come up with a highly detailed shopping list that includes quantities of food that you need.

For example, if you will be having four portions of protein per day that are four ounces each, and you want to purchase a week's worth of groceries, you know that you will need to purchase twenty-eight portions in total. This can be divided up between eggs, vegetarian substitutes, meats, and low-fat dairy options. If you plan for your shopping trip, you should have a very clear idea of exactly how much of each item you would like to purchase before you arrive at the store.

In addition to the essential supplies, there are some additional items that you may want to consider adding to your pantry including:

- Broth
- Low-fat soups
- Sugar substitutes
- Butter substitute spray
- Pan spray
- Condiments

FACT

Some people find it easier to go without something rather than use a substitute. For example, it may be preferable to go without soda altogether rather than switching to diet. The same may be true for butter substitutes, fat-free dairy products, and condiments such as mayonnaise. It is really a matter of personal preference.

Portion Control Without Leaving the Store

When you are buying meat, fish, and seafood at the grocery store, consider having each portion wrapped individually. This way you can buy a pound of meat but still cook a single portion at a time without having to thaw the entire pound or having to get out your food scale to make sure the portion is the right size.

Meat shrinks and loses moisture when cooked, so it is important to know if your portion size is a precooked weight or a cooked weight. A portion of meat can be as much as 50 percent smaller after cooking, depending on how it is cooked and how well done you like it.

Sharing Your Pantry

If you are sharing your pantry with a family or spouse, you may want to consider designating a specific shelf or cupboard for your food. This is where you can stash your healthy cereal, your whole wheat crackers, low-fat soups, and other items that are staples for your diet. This designated pantry serves two purposes. You don't have to look past the potato chips and other snacks in the house to find the nutritious items you are looking for, and you can tell at a glance if you are running low on your favorite foods.

Don't underestimate the appeal of nutritious food. Family members may not be as tempted by your whole wheat snack crackers as they are by ice cream, but that doesn't mean they won't be gone when you are looking for them.

Organizing Your Kitchen

You may find that you use your refrigerator and freezer much more than the dry storage that you relied upon in the past. As you move away from processed, canned, and shelf-stable foods and increase the amount of fresh and frozen food in your diet, your pantry may look empty compared to how it was in the past. On the other hand, your freezer may end up overflowing and your veggie bin may have more in it than ever before.

Don't Forget the Herbs and Spices

The other thing you may want to purchase is a selection of spices. If they are available in small quantities, it is much easier to use them before they lose flavor. Spices are an inexpensive way to make something unique out of some basic foods. Try using new spices that you've never tried in the past. Spices are generally inexpensive, so tossing something new in your cart won't break the bank and may help you pump up the flavor of your food.

ESSENTIAL

Many spice blends are now available without salt. If you are worried about your blood pressure, or just trying to decrease the amount of salt in your diet, take the time to find spices that are low in salt (often called sodium on spice labels).

Many grocery stores now offer fresh herbs, in addition to the more common dried varieties. They are typically found in the produce department, in a refrigerator case. They should be fresh in appearance, and might have some condensation in the packaging as they should be kept moist. The leaves should not be dried, yellowing with age, or discolored. Wilted leaves will also be an indication that the herbs are not as fresh as they should be.

If the fresh herbs are not so fresh, they won't be worth the added expense, and dried herbs should be substituted. If the herbs do not appear freshly picked, move on to the spice aisle.

Cleaning Out Your Pantry

It's time for the big clean out. Before you start, remember the goal isn't to throw away everything you've ever purchased that contains a gram of sugar, or a milligram of sodium. The goal is to make it possible, and potentially very easy, to prepare meals for yourself that fit with your weight loss plan. Eliminating temptation is a good idea, and just giving the kitchen a good spring cleaning of sorts will help you find what you need when you need it.

Check Expiration Dates

If it has an expiration date, check it. Even if it is a food you have a use for, if the expiration date says it is done, throw it out! Sometimes the date is hidden on the bottom of a can, or printed near the ingredient list, but it is well worth taking the time to look.

Even if there is no date, bulging cans and dented cans need to go, as do items that are freezer burned, stale, or clearly past their prime.

Read Labels

This step is a little more time consuming than just tossing the items that no longer have appeal or are expired. You need to read the label and determine if the food is appropriate for your new way of life. Is it loaded in sugar? Is it absurdly high in calories? It is full of fat? Does it have no nutritional value whatsoever? If the item is lacking in nutrition or is a food that might trigger you to overeat, consider doing one of two things: saving it for a special occasion or donating it to the food pantry.

Spices Expire

Some dry seasonings have a shelf life of only six months. While spices don't typically go bad, they do become far less flavorful. Herbs tend to last longer than spices, and airtight containers can extend the life of your seasonings significantly. You can usually tell with just a quick sniff if your herbs and spices are beyond their useful life and should be replaced. If your spices no longer have an intense scent, they are probably past their useful life.

Remove Temptation

If you live by yourself, the process of removing temptations from your kitchen may be easy to do. You know better than anyone else what foods trigger you to overeat, or foods that you know aren't an ideal part of your new way of life. Consider removing foods that are high in sugar, are low in nutrition (like potato chips, or cookies), or that may be perfectly healthy but you can't seem to stop eating after one portion.

Sharing your kitchen with a family is a bit trickier, as you may find yourself keeping foods that you would otherwise discard. While removing all less-than-desirable foods might be helpful early on, remember that junk foods are everywhere, and resisting them is more about your mindset than about not being able to see them. If your family insists on keeping some of these foods in the house, all is not lost; between your surgery and the support you will be receiving after surgery, you will probably be able to resist these items more successfully than you might expect.

It is important to remember that convenience foods like candy bars are available at gas stations, workplaces, grocery stores, and so many other places that you can never avoid them completely. Keeping favorite foods in the house shouldn't destroy your weight loss plan if you remain accountable for your eating.

ALERT

If gift baskets and other food items have a way of showing up at your house during the holidays, consider donating the items to a local food pantry, or taking the items to work, church, or another place of your choosing. Sharing your gift will be more satisfying than throwing it away and you won't have to worry about eating it yourself.

That said, if you have a weakness for a specific food or type of food, you may want to purge it from your pantry. Are you a chocoholic who can't walk by any type of chocolate without eating the whole thing? Out with the chocolate. Perhaps you intensely dislike a certain kind of snack, so it isn't a problem to have it in the house. You may consider keeping it around so your family doesn't complain about the lack of snacks in the house, as you won't be tempted in the slightest.

Grocery Shopping

Shopping for groceries should be much more fun than cleaning the pantry. Now you get to be creative, coming up with unique ways to eat in a nutritious way that is still tasty. Once you cover the basics, you can branch out into trying variations on recipes, with new spices, marinades, and more.

If you are thinking of making a switch from standard produce to organic produce, you may need to make more than one trip to meet all of your shopping needs. Farmer's markets and grocery stores that focus on natural or "health" food may make your shopping easier. Organic produce had a reputation of being significantly more expensive, but in recent years the difference in prices has become less notable. Proponents of organic eating say that organic produce tastes better, but you are the best judge of where the best produce for you can be found in your area. Proteins are also available in organic or grain-fed varieties, but again, it is a personal choice and shouldn't affect your diet if you choose more standard protein.

Aisles to Frequent and Aisles to Avoid

The diet danger lurks in the interior aisles of the supermarket for the most part, where the processed foods, boxed meals, junk food, candy, and desserts are found. The interior aisles are not completely devoid of value—cereals and whole grains including rice are found in these aisles, as are broths, soups, and canned vegetables. Just don't plan on doing the majority of your shopping in these aisles; plan on only supplementing your major purchases in them.

You can generally skip the candy and junk food aisles completely. The cookie and cracker aisle might have some redeeming items to offer but they are few and far between. The frozen food section, which typically resides at one end of the store, has some excellent offerings, but also contains frozen desserts, pizzas, and snacks, so it is important to be selective.

FACT

If you are craving a certain snack or food item, consider purchasing it and having two or three bites and discarding the rest of the portion. That way you've satisfied your craving, but you haven't harmed your diet plan. Usually, a few bites of a treat are enough to make the craving go away, but not so much that you've overdone it for the day.

Shopping from a List

If you have never shopped using a list before, this is a great time to start. You can be general about your purchases (i.e., "chicken"), or you can get very specific ("ten six-ounce portions of chicken, individually wrapped"). Studies show that people who use a list and stick to that list not only save significant amounts of money, but they tend to eat more healthfully as they ignore temptations they see in the store.

Using a list will ensure you don't forget what you need, but it can also help encourage you to try new things. If you are bored with some of your diet staples, don't hesitate to write "new marinade," "new spices," or even "new kind of fish" on your list.

Creating a Master Shopping List

If you like to shop from a list, consider making a master list of the items you like to keep on hand in your kitchen. The more detailed the list, the better, even including spices, condiments, and other less frequently purchased items. It may take a bit of time to create, but if you save it on the computer you can easily add and delete items over time. When you find a new item that you like, add it to the list.

To use your shopping list, you would just print a copy of your master list, check the things you need, and off to the store you go. You can even keep one on the refrigerator or some other place in the kitchen where you can indicate things you need as you think about them.

How Grocery Stores Are Arranged

Grocery stores are not set up to make your shopping easier, nor are they arranged to help you stick to your diet plan. A grocery store is arranged for one specific purpose: to make you spend more money. Everything from the placement of food on the shelves to how the different departments are arranged are based on how well they achieve the objective of getting you to place items in your cart.

Take for example the cereal aisle. The least expensive, and typically the most nutritious cereals, are typically on the highest shelves and the very lowest shelves, where you are the least likely to notice them. On the center shelves, where children can see them easily and where you are most likely to notice them, are the more expensive, high-sugar, low-fiber-content cereals in the bright boxes to catch your eye.

In the majority of grocery stores, the fundamentals of your diet will be located on the perimeter of the store. This is where you will find dairy items, the meat counter, the produce section, and the bread section. If you stick to these areas when purchasing your food, read the labels on your dairy selections and breads, and make a point to choose lower-fat proteins, you will be making solid choices for your diet.

How to Choose the Best Protein

Since protein will be a key ingredient in your diet plan you'll need to know what to look for when shopping. Fresh meat should look moist and fresh. It often has a sheen that indicates that there is moisture both in and on the meat. The color should be bright, but not too bright; often fish that is a bright pink color has been treated to look fresher and more appealing. If meat is starting to look dry or take on a brown or gray cast around the edges, it isn't as fresh as it should be. If you are looking at beef, there should be minimal marbling, or fat streaking. The more streaking, the higher the fat content. Fat around the edges of the cut is less concerning as you can remove it prior to cooking.

Ground beef may be slightly brown as it is exposed to the air, but should not look dried on the edges. Look for "extra lean," which is often designated as 96/4 or 94/6, meaning that the meat has 4 or 6 percent fat content. Meat at the counter will not typically have labels that give you nutritional information such as fat content, so you may want a nutrition guide/calorie count book that allows you to look up information on the food you are considering buying.

ALERT

If you are thinking of buying a whole fish, look at the eyes of the fish. Are they bright and shiny? The gills should still be pink or even red, and there should be an appearance of moisture without being slimy.

Last-Minute Cart Check

Once you put food in your cart and head to the checkout area, there is no grocery law that prevents you from examining your purchases and taking things out of the cart. When you are waiting in line to be checked out, or even when you think you've gotten everything you need, and maybe more, look over what you are planning to buy.

Are the foods you are buying a nutritious addition to your diet, or are you starting to slip into old habits that aren't part of your weight loss plan? Are you strictly adhering to your surgeon's suggestions, or are you starting to slip old habits back into your diet? This last-minute cart check can help you get back on track before you ever really go off track, just by preventing you from taking food home that you really don't need.

Reading Labels

If you have food allergies or are particular about your groceries, you may already be a die-hard label reader. If you aren't, this is the time to begin reading the labels of everything you purchase. There are multiple reasons for this, including hidden fat, sodium, and sugar, along with how many calories are contained in the food.

It is remarkable how many items contain unexpected ingredients. Ketchup, for example, typically contains a large amount of sugar, as does tomato sauce. Many soups can be very high in fat and even higher in sodium, even when they are vegetarian.

One thing to remember when reading labels is that portion sizes vary widely. A single can may have one serving or five, which makes an enormous difference when trying to determine how many calories you are eating.

Misleading Labels

Labels can be misleading, and often the more detailed they are, the more closely they need to be read. The wide variety of terms used to promote foods are not always clear. "Reduced fat," for example, doesn't necessarily mean the item is low in fat, it just means that it has 25 percent less fat in it than the food it is being compared to. The same is true of "reduced sodium" items, which may still have significant amounts of sodium.

Sugar Content

"Sugar-free" foods are not absolutely sugar free. These foods contain less than .5 grams per serving. No-added-sugar foods can still be high in sugar if the original food was high in sugar. For example, mandarin oranges in a can may still contain natural sugars, but no additional sugar was added in the canning process.

Calorie Content

"Calorie free" means that a serving of the food has less than five calories. Be sure to check portion sizes, as the portion required to be calorie-free may be so small as to be ridiculous. "Low-calorie" foods contain forty calories or less per serving.

Fat Content

"Fat free" on a label indicates that a serving has less than a half gram of fat per serving, while "saturated fat free" means that there is less than a half gram of saturated fat per serving, but there may be additional unsaturated fat in each serving. An item that is "saturated fat free" could potentially be low in saturated fats but still brimming with total fat. "Low fat" means three grams of fat or less per serving.

Sodium Content

"Sodium-free" foods contain 5 milligrams or less per serving, and low-sodium foods have 140 milligrams or less. "Very low-sodium" items have 35 milligrams or less per serving and "less" sodium indicates at least 25 percent less sodium than the comparison food.

Fiber Content

A "high-fiber" food offers no less than 5 grams of fiber per serving, while a label stating "good source of fiber" must have 2.5 to 4.9 grams in a serving. "Added fiber" or "more fiber" indicates that there are 2.5 grams more fiber in every serving than in the comparison food.

Serving Sizes

Serving sizes vary widely from can to can. A twelve-ounce can of soup may have two servings, while the same size can of a different type of soup may have four servings. If you are trying to compare products, make sure the comparison is a fair one. Bread is often very hard to compare, as one loaf may give a serving size as one slice of bread, while another may indicate three slices of bread.

Organic Food

The "certified organic" label means that the food was grown without chemical fertilizer, herbicides, pesticides, or hormones. In addition, the ground on which the food was grown cannot have been exposed to those agents in the last seven years. If meat is labeled as organic, the pastures on which they were raised have been chemical free for the last seven years and they were not fed grain or other foods that are not organic.

Products made of multiple ingredients can be labeled "100 percent organic"; "organic," which means 95 percent organic content; or "made with organic ingredients," which means no less than 70 percent organic ingredients. Obtaining organic certification is very expensive, so even farms that qualify for organic status may not label their food as "organic" because they cannot afford to submit to the official process.

CHAPTER 11

How to Cook after Weight Loss Surgery

Cooking for yourself is one of the best things you can do after having weight loss surgery. Cooking your own food puts you in control, allowing you to use fresh ingredients, decide upon portion sizes, and limit how much fat, salt, and sugar is added. Cooking for yourself can be pleasurable, and while it certainly isn't as quick and easy as ordering from a menu, with some thought and planning, cooking at home does not need to be a burden.

Ideal Cooking Techniques

While cooking for yourself puts you in control of what you are making, it isn't necessarily enough to have a positive impact on your weight loss. In order to truly be compliant with your new eating plan, you will need to choose what you cook and how you cook more carefully than you may have in the past.

You may have to adapt recipes that you've enjoyed in the past to make them appropriate for your new way of life, but in many cases it is far easier to seek out new recipes and look for things that are both appealing and in line with your new dietary needs. This doesn't mean you'll never be able to have that favorite food again, but you may have to postpone having it, or make it a special "holidays only" treat.

When cooking, it may take a concerted effort not to pour oil into a pan before cooking, just as it might be difficult to avoid the sugar bowl when having your morning coffee.

Baking

Baking is probably not new territory to you, but baking without making cheesy casseroles or adding fat may be less familiar. Nonstick cookie sheets or bakeware will make it easier to cook your proteins without adding oil, as the coating will prevent your food from sticking even if you don't use a single drop of oil.

ESSENTIAL

Combining sautéing with baking can produce wonderfully moist protein dishes. Start cooking your chicken by quickly sautéing it on both sides in an oven-safe sauté pan. Once both sides are lightly browned, finish cooking the chicken in the oven. Searing the outside of the meat keeps the moisture in, and baking cooks the meat without making it tough.

You may also want to consider purchasing a baking stone, which helps foods become crisp while baking, or a vented cookie sheet, which also promotes crisping. Baking is appropriate for all types of proteins and can also be used for most vegetables.

Broiling

"Broiling" is just a fancy term for cooking by exposing the food to direct heat. Barbecuing is one type of broiling, but you do not need a grill to broil food. Most ovens have a broiler inside that allows you to cook quickly at high temperatures. The downside of broiling is that if you aren't paying attention, you may end up with a meal that looks more like a charcoal briquette than a tempting piece of fish.

Broiling is great for a low fat-diet for several reasons. The high temperatures quickly sear the meat, locking in moisture for a more moist and tender meal. Broiling requires no fat to be tasty, but can be greatly enhanced by a spice rub or marinade. Broiling can also be used for vegetables, and even starches, such as broiled potatoes.

If you have a barbecue grill, broiling can be quick and easy and requires minimal cleanup. Even crab legs can be cooked on the grill, so don't hesitate to fire your grill up to cook a meal. If you use charcoal, or add aromatic hardwoods to your fire, this type of broiling will enhance most flavors.

Poaching

"Poaching" just means to cook by placing the food in a simmering liquid. You may have had poached eggs in the past, but poaching in water is just the tip of the iceberg. Fruit, such as pears, can be poached in fruit juice, and fish can be poached in a broth that adds flavor with minimal calories.

If you plan to poach food, the water should be at a simmer, which means it is hot enough to be moving slightly, but not so hot that it is bubbling.

Simmer

Simmering is a method of cooking that doesn't quite reach the boiling point. If you are heating a can of soup, you probably heat the soup until it simmers prior to serving it. A simmer is not quite as hot as boiling, and is frequently used for sauces, broths, and soups. When you are heating and cooking foods on the stove, you are most often using a simmer, so cooking with this method should not be difficult.

Ideally, if you would like to simmer your food, the temperature should be hot enough that the liquids bubble occasionally, but not rapidly.

Boiling

Boiling is a great way to cook some foods with a minimum of effort and no added calories. Boiled eggs are great, rice should be boiled, and pasta certainly wouldn't be the same if it wasn't thrown into a pot of boiling water before serving. The uses of boiling are somewhat limited, though, because boiling vegetables tends to cause a loss of vitamins and minerals into the water, and it can result in some very bland foods.

Potatoes can be boiled, certainly, but tend to taste better when baked or roasted.

If you plan to boil your food, the water in the pan should be bubbling constantly, known as a "full boil" or bubbling vigorously, also known as a "rolling boil."

ESSENTIAL

Add flavor to your boiled foods by adding herbs and spices to the water. You may want to try adding a spice blend of your own to the boiling pot, or a premade one that is low in sodium. Something as simple as dried onions or garlic can add a considerable amount of flavor to your food.

Steaming

Steaming is the method of cooking with heated water vapor. Unlike boiling, the food doesn't come into direct contact with the hot water, just the vapor from it, so minimal nutrients are lost from this method. Steaming is the ideal way to cook vegetables, as there are no added calories. Steaming can also bring out the bright, natural colors of vegetables, and it can be done with flavorful liquids such as broths rather than just water.

Wrapping

Wrapping is just what it sounds like, wrapping a food and then cooking it in the wrapper to enhance the flavor. Wrappers vary widely, and include paper and organic material. Some cooks prefer to use parchment paper to make a paper envelope, then place fish or another protein in the envelope, along with herbs, spices, and even vegetables. The envelope is then baked, allowing the protein to cook, bake, or steam while absorbing new flavors. Other types of wrapping include using banana leaves and grape leaves.

Braise

Braising is a cooking method that is typically used for meats that need to be cooked very slowly in order to be tender. The meat is typically seared on both sides, then placed in a pan with a small amount of liquid, covered, and cooked over low heat until so tender it falls apart with a fork.

Cuts of meat that are lower in fat tend to be less tender, as do less expensive pieces of meat, so this cooking method is ideal for both. A roast is an excellent example of a meat that can be braised to bring out the best texture, without requiring additional oil.

Searing

Searing is a method that uses very high heat to cook the outside of proteins rapidly. Searing isn't typically used to cook the food in its entirety, rather it is just a way to brown the outside of the meat and to seal in moisture and flavor.

To sear a piece of meat, the pan must be very hot, and before adding the meat, add a small amount of stock or broth. Place the meat in the pan, turning over after a few minutes, to sear both sides. Once the meat has been browned, finish cooking in the oven or at a lower temperature on the stove.

Cooking a piece of meat using the searing technique exclusively can result in a very tough piece of meat, so plan on finishing the meat with slow cooking, braising, or baking.

Slow Cooking

There is little difference between braising and slow cooking when it comes to meat, but slow cooking applies to other foods as well. A slow cooker, commonly known as a Crock-Pot, is designed to cook a variety of foods at low temperatures for extended periods of time. This method is ideal for soups and stews, tenderizing meats, and cooking vegetables slowly.

Like braising, flavorful liquids can be used, rather than plain water. Broth and stocks, along with herbs and spices, can improve the flavor of slow-cooked foods, without adding too many additional calories.

Sauté

Sautéing means to cook quickly with oil in a hot pan. Sautéing isn't necessarily bad, but it can be, depending upon the amount of oil used. Minimal oil is necessary to sauté; a teaspoon is plenty in many cases, but most people use significantly more.

If you are going to sauté, measure the amount of oil you use to prevent adding too much fat and too many calories to your meal. Make sure the pan is hot prior to adding the oil, then add your food.

Easy Substitutions

Your favorite foods and recipes need not be eliminated from your life if they can be easily adapted to your new eating style. Some of these fixes are quick and easy, while others may require some experimentation. You may discover substitutions on your own that work to convert recipes that you enjoy.

One of the easiest substitutions you can make is just to purchase a lower-fat version of the same item. For example, instead of buying full-fat sour cream, try a reduced-fat or fat-free version. Instead of soft drinks with hundreds of empty calories from sugar, switch to a diet version that has no calories.

Egg Substitute

Eggs are generally a healthy option, but if you are concerned about your fat intake, or you are battling high cholesterol, you might want to consider a substitute for whole eggs. A pasteurized egg substitute, usually found in the same section as regular eggs, is a bit of a misnomer, as they are actually made from egg whites. They look like scrambled eggs before they are cooked, and look and cook nearly identically to beaten eggs.

If you are baking, you can substitute two egg whites for a whole egg, or a quarter cup of egg substitute.

Sugar Substitutes

There are many acceptable sugar substitutes on the market that can sweeten drinks in place of real sugar. While eliminating sugar from your diet without substitutions is more desirable, it isn't always possible. Equal, Sweet N'Low, Splenda, and other brands of low- or no-calorie sweeteners are easily available. You may prefer one brand over another, so you might want to try different types of sweeteners to determine which one is best.

If you are baking, Splenda is your ideal substitute for sugar. Splenda is substituted one-to-one for sugar, and works in the vast majority of baking applications. It won't caramelize like real sugar, browning under heat, but it does provide the sweetness needed for sugar-free cakes, brownies, and other sweets.

Fat Substitutes for Baking

If your favorite baked good calls for oil, you may be able to substitute an equal amount of applesauce for the oil. Most fruit purees will work, but some are sweeter than others, so unsweetened applesauce may work better for a lightly sweet baked good, while a prune puree may be better for a much sweeter item.

If the item you are baking is more savory, such as bread, you can substitute up to half of the fat the recipe calls for with fat-free or low-fat buttermilk or yogurt in a two-to-one ratio. For example, if a recipe calls for a cup of oil, you would use a half cup of oil and a quarter cup of buttermilk. If the batter looks overly dry, you can add additional buttermilk until the batter is the proper consistency.

Fat Substitutes When Cooking Protein

When cooking a piece of meat, it may be your habit to put oil in the bottom of the pan. With a good nonstick pan, oil isn't necessary to prevent meat from sticking, but that won't help with the flavor lost from cooking without fat.

To help enhance flavor without using butter or oil, consider putting broth or stock in the bottom of the pan. You can also try a variety of herbs and spices, including a rub or a marinade, prior to putting the meat in the pan.

Mayonnaise Substitutes

There are a number of ways to eliminate mayonnaise for a variety of purposes. If you are accustomed to putting mayonnaise on a sandwich and want to eliminate the fat, consider trying a low fat creamy salad dressing. If you are making a pasta salad that calls for mayonnaise, consider substituting low-fat sour cream or plain yogurt. The same substitution is appropriate if you are trying to make a low-fat salad dressing.

Ground Meat Substitutes

If you are craving tacos but dread the fat that is usually found in ground beef, all is not lost. There are multiple ways to prepare ground meats that reduce the fat content but keep the flavor. It is important to start out with the leanest meat possible; for example, ground chuck is 20 percent fat, but some ground beef has as little as 4 percent fat.

Once you have lean meat, there are additional ways to decrease the overall fat content. You can use an extender, such as oatmeal, adding it to the meat to increase the amount of bulk without adding fat. This is a common approach when making a meat loaf or meatballs, because it creates a more smooth texture.

Another way to make ground meats a healthier option is to use more than one type of ground meat. A mixture of half ground beef and half ground chicken isn't notably different in many recipes than using just ground beef. Ground turkey can also be used for this purpose, but it tends to be dry, so it should be used in smaller quantities than other ground meats.

Texturized Vegetable Protein, or TVP, is a vegetarian substitute for meat. It comes as a hard nugget, in a variety of shapes, and is used by vegetarians to add protein to their meatless diets. TVP has to be reconstituted, or rehydrated, by soaking with hot water. TVP can also be added to ground meats to lower the fat content while increasing the protein content. A small amount of TVP can be added to a mixture of ground beef without making a notable difference, and is a secret ingredient in many fast food burgers and tacos.

Cooking Techniques and Foods to Avoid

To make it easier to find new recipes and foods that you can prepare yourself, it is essential to start out with a discussion of what is no longer appropriate when cooking for yourself. It may seem like a no-brainer to eliminate deep fat frying from your culinary repertoire, but many other preparations aren't so obvious in the hazards they present for your diet.

Candied

If you are sensitive to dumping syndrome, candied food should be avoided at all costs, and for those who aren't sensitive to sugar in that way, candying is still not an ideal preparation. Typically done by tossing fruit or vegetables with a combination of hot butter and melted sugar, candying can add a tremendous amount of fat and calories to your otherwise healthy produce.

Fried

Fried doesn't just include throwing food into a deep fryer. Preparations to avoid include pan-frying, deep frying, stir frying, and even sautéing if a large quantity of oil is required. It doesn't matter if you are using unsaturated fat or saturated fat, butter or oil, shortening or margarine. Frying gives food an opportunity to absorb far more oil than most people realize; it's not just resting on the outside of the food.

Wondering if a food is fried? Look for words like "crispy" or "crunchy." Fruit and vegetables can be crunchy and crispy without oil, but most other foods cannot.

With a whopping 100 calories or more per tablespoon, frying can pack on the fat and calories, not to mention helping to maintain high cholesterol levels. Small quantities of oils are certainly acceptable, to coat the pan or a spritz for flavor, or as part of a marinade, but larger quantities should be avoided whenever possible.

Creamy and Cheesy

Cream and cheese can take a perfectly healthy diet option like chicken and make it a diet buster extraordinaire. Both cream and cheese disguise themselves under a variety of names, including Alfredo sauce, butter sauce, Piccata, whipped cream, cream cheese, Parmesan-crusted, cream-based, and other descriptions.

If you are cooking for yourself or eating in a restaurant, phrases like "a light butter sauce" should set off alarm bells in your head. A butter sauce can only be light in comparison to a lard sauce, so don't let terms like "light," "reduced-calorie," or "diet-friendly" fool you into making a poor choice.

If you are trying to decide upon a recipe to try, look for one that doesn't include cream, cheese, butter, lard, margarine, oil, shortening, or other calorie- and fat-dense ingredients. These items have a strong tendency to ruin an otherwise healthful dish. Take for example broccoli. Perfectly healthy when steamed, not so much so when topped with a cheese sauce.

Baked Sweets

With the addition of sweeteners like Splenda that can be used in baking, a cake doesn't have to be a diet disaster, but sweets in general should be considered a once-in-a-great-while food. Desserts in general are bad for your plan for two reasons: They typically include refined flour with little nutritional value, and they almost always have a huge amount of refined white sugar to make them sweet.

While the sugar in most desserts can be replaced with a low- or no-calorie sweetener, the empty calories remain. Even worse, if you begin to substitute "healthy" sweets for the items you used to eat, you may never lose your taste for sugar. Keep in mind that some studies show that adding sugar alternatives to your diet may increase your craving for sweets, so even adapted sweets should be eaten in moderation.

As your tastes begin to change, especially if you eliminate most sugar from your diet, you may be pleasantly surprised at how fruit starts to become an acceptable dessert. The sweetness will be more pronounced and seem more dessert-like than it may have in the past.

Crusted, Battered, and Stuffed

A chicken breast can be a beautiful thing, until you put a crust on it, or stuff it, among other things. If you are putting a crust on your protein by dredging it in a flour preparation, or filling a pork chop with stuffing, there is a high likelihood that your healthy piece of meat has just tripled in calories. Putting a crust on your protein isn't necessarily a bad thing, and it can be done in a reasonable fashion that is healthful, but use caution and carefully evaluate how you are doing it. If you are whipping up a batter, dipping your protein and frying it until crispy, you're in a bad diet place.

Another kind of crust is equally bad in terms of fat and calories: the pie crust. Crusts come in a variety of forms, including puff pastry, some pizza dough, and pie dough, none of which are healthy additions to your meal. If you are craving something that normally comes with a crust, consider making it without the crust, such as a crustless potpie, or using an alternative crust. For example, making a pizza on a large whole-grain tortilla can be tasty, just as a mini pizza on a bagel or English muffin can be a great treat. Phyllo dough, which is fat free, makes a great top crust on dishes where you want a crust but don't want the calories.

FACT

If you crave a crust on your protein but you know that battering and deep frying is a bad thing, consider tossing the protein (such as chicken) in beaten egg whites, then rolling it in low-fat bread crumbs such as Panko. Baking it will make it crispy without the fat of frying.

Essentials for Cooking

If you aren't someone who enjoyed cooking in the past, or even if you are an accomplished cook who needs to modify what and how you cook, there are some things that your kitchen may need. A few small purchases, along with a well-planned grocery shopping trip, can make it much easier to prepare meals that comply with your diet.

Nonstick Cookware

A great nonstick pan can completely eliminate the need for oil in the pan to prevent food from sticking. Investing in at least one pan with a professional-grade nonstick coating will allow you to cook all of your proteins, such as chicken or pork, without the addition of a drop of oil.

Nonstick pans aren't just helpful for cooking proteins, fresh vegetables can be quickly sautéed with broth or minimal oil and tossed easily when you aren't struggling to prevent them from adhering to the bottom of the pan.

Food Steamers

A steamer will be a valuable addition to your kitchen. You need not go out and purchase a stand-alone steamer with a timer to have an effective steamer. There are compact steamers that can be placed in a microwave, sauce pan inserts that turn any basic pan into a steamer, and even bamboo steamers that allow you to steam multiple foods on separate layers of the steamer.

Steaming will help you cook proteins such as eggs (poaching, or in place of boiling) with no added fat, and with the addition of herbs and spices, it can result in tasty vegetables with a minimum of effort.

Nonfat Cooking Spray

A nonfat cooking spray can be very helpful when trying to cook without added fat. Cooking sprays come in an aerosol can, allowing you to spray tiny amounts onto your food or pan. If you prefer to use your own oil, hand pump containers are available that allow you to spray your oil of choice into a pan or onto a salad.

FACT

Cooking sprays have improved dramatically in recent years. They are now available in flavors as well as filled with different oils such as olive oil. If you would like to use more unique oils, such as hazelnut, sesame, or peanut oil, consider buying your own oil sprayer, which allows you to use most types of oils as you would use cooking spray.

The benefit from spray oils is that the portion size used to lightly cover your food is significantly less than what you would use to toss your food in oil or when dressing a salad. A quick mist of oil provides the flavor you are looking for, but without the large quantities of oil you want to avoid.

Colanders and Strainers

Colanders are kitchen staples for many reasons. They can be used to drain water from pasta, to remove the water from your steaming vegetables, and many other purposes. If you have a colander with a fine enough mesh, you can also use them to strain your ground beef. Rather than retaining the fat that comes out of ground beef and incorporating it into your food, you can toss the ground beef and strain the excess oil. If you feel that isn't adequate, you can even rinse the meat with hot water to remove additional fat. Don't rinse too long, just a quick rinse in hot water, or the meat may get mushy.

Measuring Devices

Measuring and weighing your food will be essential to your successful weight loss. It is too easy to underestimate portion sizes and calorie content if you aren't taking the time to precisely measure the size of your servings. An extra ounce or two of meat might not seem like it is worth worrying about, but when multiplied over dozens or hundreds of meals, the difference can be significant.

Plan on measuring everything you eat, when possible, for the first few months after your procedure. This includes beverages with calories, vegetables, and anything else that doesn't come in a single serving, such as a piece of bread. Over time, you will become adept at estimating portion sizes at a glance. Even when you've become an expert portion controller, it is still a good idea to measure your food for a day every few weeks, to make sure you're as accurate as you'd like to be.

You'll need, at the minimum, an accurate food scale, a set of measuring cups, and a set of measuring spoons. If you are someone who enjoys cooking, you may want to purchase measuring cups in a variety of sizes and styles, as some come with pouring spouts, and others are easier to use with dry ingredients.

Portions

Once you've cooked a delicious meal, it is easy to forget one of the most important parts of cooking for yourself: portion control. Most of the information available about nutrition and how much you should be eating of each food group won't be appropriate for you. A cup of broccoli might be a "normal" portion, but when your entire meal is only half a cup to a cup in size, that portion will be far too large.

Your surgeon should provide information about how much you should be eating of each food group throughout the day. These portions will change as you move through the stages of recovery and adapt to your new lifestyle.

One of the easiest ways to control your portions is to portion foods when you get home from the grocery store or after cooking. For example, if you buy a large quantity of chicken breasts to save money, you can grab your food scale, cut each breast into the appropriate portions, and put it into the refrigerator or freezer. That way, when it is time to cook, whether for yourself or your entire family, you can quickly cook appropriate portions without a great deal of fuss.

Making portion control simple will help you stick with appropriate portion sizes. When portion control becomes a giant hassle, it is much easier to ignore. If you are someone who is always running late in the morning, but you want to pack your lunch, consider portioning your salad out and placing it in containers ready for work when you get home from the grocery store. Another way to make portion control easy is to purchase prepackaged and appropriately portioned foods. If you are going to have dairy in your lunch, consider individually wrapped string cheese, or individual servings of cottage cheese.

CHAPTER 12

Breaking Through a Weight Loss Plateau

A weight loss plateau is not something weight loss patients look forward to having, but if you reach one, it doesn't necessarily mean that you won't reach your goals. Learn more about plateaus, including some of the causes, why it may not really be a plateau at all, and most importantly, what you can do to break through yours.

Weight Loss Plateaus

A weight loss plateau is typically described as two or more weeks without weight loss. For those trying to lose weight, the term does not adequately describe the frustration that is felt when the pounds stop coming off. There are many reasons that a plateau may happen, but don't despair; there are many ways to get back on track and get the scale moving in the right direction again.

Before you get upset about the lack of weight loss, it is important to know that a plateau is often a normal part of weight loss. It is possible to do all the right things and still experience a slowdown in your results. A week or two without a loss isn't necessarily cause for alarm, it may just be your body's way of settling into your new regime. When a plateau stretches past the two-week mark, however, it is time to evaluate what you are doing on a daily and weekly basis.

If you are experiencing a plateau, don't panic. You could be experiencing water retention, it may be a week where you are losing inches rather than pounds, or even something as simple as wearing different clothing than the last time you weighed yourself.

Evaluate Your Routine

If you've experienced two weeks without weight loss, it is time to examine your daily and weekly routines. Unfortunately, one bad day can erase many days of hard work and proper nutrition, so it is important to look at what you are doing as a whole, rather than a day at a time. If you have been doing very well Monday through Friday, but tend to consume many calories on the weekend in the form of food or drink, you may need to change those habits to get back on track. Perfection in your diet is not a realistic expectation, but if you are routinely sabotaging several days' worth of effort, you will need to get to the root of the problem to change it.

It isn't enough to eat properly if you want to be a highly successful weight loss surgery patient. In the early months, altering your diet alone can produce amazing results, but in the long term, exercise is absolutely essential if you want to reach your goal weight and maintain the loss. If you haven't started exercising, now is the time to start.

What Are You Doing Right?

Before you get too focused on the things that may be hindering your weight loss, take the time to think about what you are doing right. More than likely, your positive changes since your surgery outweigh any negatives. You've probably made great strides in altering the way you approach meal times, cooking, and snacking. You may have eliminated sugar from your diet, along with junk food and fast food.

It is important that you acknowledge all of the things you are doing well! Congratulate yourself for all of the hard work you have done to get to this point. Remember, you can't have a plateau if you weren't losing weight to begin with, so you've already found some level of success.

What Are You Doing Wrong?

Before you start to really evaluate your routine and determine where you can do a better job working toward your goal weight, find the written dietary instructions that your surgeon provided. They should list, in great detail, what you should be eating, how much you should be eating, and when you should be eating.

ESSENTIAL

When you are evaluating your bad habits, try not to be too hard on yourself. The idea is to see where you can make improvements, not to make yourself feel bad about what you are doing. Try to be positive about the changes you can make, for example: "In the future I will drink less calories," and not "I'm always going to be fat, I can't seem to get it through my head that I need to stop drinking calories."

Have you strayed from those guidelines in the weeks and months since your surgery? Are you finding yourself snacking even though you know you should be eating three full meals with little or nothing in between? Are you eating foods that contain little nutrition but are high in calories?

Here are some questions to ask yourself:

- How closely am I following the surgeon's dietary guidelines?
- Am I drinking calories?

- Am I skipping meals?
- Am I getting away from the portion size I used at the beginning of the process?
- Am I exercising regularly?
- Am I doing things on the weekend that erase the progress I made during the week?
- Am I eating because of "brain hunger" instead of "stomach hunger"?
- Am I eating past the point of feeling full?
- Am I eating foods that are not nutritious, or foods that trigger cravings?
- Am I cooking for myself so that I know exactly what is in my food?
- Am I eating dinner in restaurants too often?
- Am I drinking enough water?
- Am I drinking water when I shouldn't?
- Am I drinking alcohol too frequently?
- Am I weighing and measuring portions, or just guessing?
- Are fatty, high-calorie foods such as butter sneaking into my foods?
- Are sugary gum, candies, mints, and other small treats part of my diet?
- How many calories am I eating each day?
- Am I eating the recommended amount of protein each day?
- What can I do better?

Take a good look at what you are doing to actively continue losing weight. You may find that you are doing many of the right things and that with a few small changes you will be back on track and losing weight steadily. You may also find that you've strayed away from your initial diet plan without even realizing it. Going back to your surgeon's guidelines will help jump-start your weight loss and get you on track.

In some cases, you may even find that you are doing the right things and there isn't much that you should change.

As you lose weight you may need to adjust your calorie intake. This is especially true if you are nearing your goal weight or if you haven't adjusted your daily calories even though you've been losing consistently. For example, let's say that you started out weighing 200 pounds and you lose weight as long as you only eat 8 calories for every pound of your body weight. At 200 pounds, you could eat 1,400 calories a day and still lose weight. However, at 175 pounds, 8 calories per pound would mean that you are eating enough calories to maintain your body weight.

Don't plan on altering your caloric intake without consulting with your surgeon. It may be preferable to burn more calories through exercise than to eat less food, or you may be tempted to be too restrictive. You don't want to consume so few calories that you are hungry all the time, as constant hunger can lead to binges and a slowing of your metabolism.

Approaching Your Goal Weight

As you approach your goal weight, you will find that your weight loss slows down. Whereas you may have lost pounds almost effortlessly in the initial few weeks after your surgery, it may take real effort to obtain much smaller results as you continue to lose weight. This is completely normal and should be expected.

You may also find that you actually gain small amounts of weight, but your clothes are getting bigger at the same time, especially if you are doing weight training or other types of exercise that build muscle. In this case, the way your clothes fit and your measurements will be a far more accurate indicator of your progress than the scale.

ESSENTIAL

Is the thought of your goal weight hindering your progress? While an ambitious goal can be a great thing, if you find yourself frustrated by your progress, or intimidated by the enormity of the challenge before you, start with mini goals. Start with "I'd like to lose another 5 pounds," rather than "I need to lose 120 pounds to get to my goal weight."

Normal Slowdown

It cannot be stressed enough that a slowdown or complete stop in weight loss that lasts a week or two is normal for most dieters. If you keep a food and exercise diary, you may want to also keep track of your menstrual periods and weight loss at the same time. You might find that your weight loss slows every month during a certain week, then picks back up again.

You may find specific foods will trigger a short-term plateau. For example, if you eat foods that are high in salt content, you may find that your fingers are swollen and you feel bloated the next day or two, meaning that you are retaining more water than usual. Retaining water can contribute to temporary gains of several pounds overnight.

Keep in mind that your weight loss will happen fastest during the six months immediately following your surgery. After that, you can expect the weight to continue to come off, but it will be at a slower rate and may require more effort to maintain momentum.

FACT

You may continue to lose the same percentage of your body weight, but it can feel like you've slowed down dramatically. For example, if your starting weight was 300 pounds, losing 1 percent of your body weight in one week meant that you were losing 3 pounds. When you are down to 150 pounds, you would only lose 1.5 pounds per week. Same rate of loss, different number of pounds.

Food Diary

Your food diary will be your best friend if you are looking for patterns of behavior or nutritional issues that are affecting your weight loss. If you started to plateau the first week of January, it will be easy to look and see if you overindulged on New Year's, or if you are seeing the results of too many Christmas cookies. You should consider doing a serious analysis of your food diary, calculating not only how many calories you are consuming but how much protein, carbohydrates, and fat you are taking in. You will also be able to count the calories that you are drinking in the form of alcohol, soda, or any other beverages.

If you keep your food diary up to date religiously, you should be able to calculate exactly how many calories you are consuming each day, along with how many grams of protein you are eating. Compare your recent weeks with the first few weeks you were eating a full diet after surgery and with the diet guidelines you were given. Are you eating the way your surgeon intended? Are you slipping back into old habits?

If you aren't measuring your food before you eat, you may have a problem that your food diary won't reveal: a slow but steady increase in portion sizes over time. Your protein serving may have grown from four ounces to six or seven ounces and you may not even realize it.

The Primary Culprits Behind a Plateau

It's official, you're experiencing a plateau. You haven't lost an ounce for two weeks, perhaps longer, but you are not at your goal weight. Some things are more likely than others to be sabotaging your efforts, whether you are close to your goal or not.

What were your worst nutritional habits before your surgery? Were you a sugar addict? A chocoholic? Perhaps you were a snacker, or you didn't need to be hungry to eat. Maybe you had trouble stopping when you were full and felt the urge to clean your plate no matter how stuffed you felt.

Think about your bad habits before surgery and take a long and honest look at what you are doing today. Are those habits creeping back into your life?

Protein Power

Emphasize protein in your diet. Most surgeons recommend that you include no less than sixty grams of protein in your diet each day. If you have reached a plateau, you should make sure you have been eating an adequate amount of protein. If you are getting enough protein, consider increasing the percentage of your diet that is comprised of protein.

Be sure to add lean protein to your diet, such as lean meats, nuts, and low-fat dairy products. There are many sources of protein that are very high in fat, so it is important to be selective when increasing your protein intake.

Eating Too Little?

It is possible to eat too few calories after weight loss surgery. It can happen if you are ill, or if you have complications after surgery, but some patients intentionally eat too few calories, thinking it will speed their weight loss.

Unfortunately, decreasing your calorie intake too much can backfire, leading to feeling lethargic and tired, and slowing your metabolism and weight loss. If you are eating less than your surgeon recommends, and you've reached a plateau, eating too little may be part of the problem. Seriously consider talking to your doctor about your eating habits and if you should add additional calories to your daily diet.

Snacking

Snacking is one of the worst things you can do as a weight loss patient. Occasional low-calorie snacks when you are truly hungry is one thing, but regular snacking can derail your progress, and even worse, lead to the return of some very bad habits. Focus on three meals a day, each with protein, fresh fruits, and vegetables and some whole grains. If you must snack, stick with fresh fruits and vegetables and keep your snack size small.

FACT

While snacking is not preferable, if you are hungry, eat! Waiting until you are absolutely starving before you eat can lead to overeating. While snacking shouldn't become a habit, if it takes the edge off and allows you to eat a reasonable meal without overindulging, have a small and healthy snack.

Calories Count

Your overall calorie count matters. In the grand scheme of things, the number of calories you consume is more important than the size of your portions, whether you drink your calories or chew them, or whether you consume more protein or more carbs. While all of those things are important, if you are consuming too many calories, it won't matter what form they take. Too many calories will mean no weight loss, or even worse, weight gain.

Keep track of the number of calories that you eat, down to the smallest nibbles, in your food diary. Keeping track of what you eat will help you stay accountable for your food consumption. It will also help you adjust your calorie consumption as you lose weight to keep the momentum going.

The Little Calories That Count

Let's say you are a coffee person. You won't get out of bed or start the day without a fresh and hot cup of coffee. You've tried nondairy creamers, low-fat cream substitutes, and a variety of other things, but you can't stand to have your coffee with anything but two tablespoons of half-and-half. Big deal right? What does that little dash of cream mean in the grand scheme of things? Well, it can mean a lot if you don't keep track of it and compensate for it in other ways.

There are forty calories in two tablespoons of half-and-half, which is not an extraordinary amount, but it can add up over time. It can add up very quickly if you are having multiple cups of coffee, but either way, it does add up. In the course of a year, one cup of coffee with two tablespoons of half-and-half will add over 14,000 calories to your diet. Do you absolutely need to remove half-and-half from your diet? No. Here's the trick: Instead of depriving yourself of the things you truly love, whether it is half-and-half in your coffee or an occasional snack, plan on compensating for your indulgence with exercise. Instead of feeling deprived and drinking coffee that you don't enjoy, plan on spending an extra ten minutes at the gym walking on a treadmill, or taking your dog for a quick walk while you sip your coffee.

Being a weight loss surgery patient doesn't mean you need to deprive yourself of all the foods you truly enjoy; it just means you need to figure out ways to make your plan accommodate the occasional indulgence.

Refined Food Versus Whole Foods

If your weight loss has stopped, it is worth looking at the things you are eating, not just for calorie content but to see if you have strayed away from whole, natural foods. Have you started eating more processed foods from boxes and cans? Are you finding yourself eating more white sugar and breads that are not whole grain?

If you are eating more food that is less nutritious, you will find that you are getting less nutrition for every calorie that you consume, and typically, feeling far less full. Getting those fresh vegetables, fruits, and whole grains back in your diet can help in a number of ways. They are high in fiber, which helps you feel full longer and prevents constipation. You can typically have a larger meal for the same number of calories, and most importantly, your meals will have far more nutritional value than the processed alternatives.

You will find that eating at restaurants will make it harder to choose whole foods, unless you stick with salads. It is an unfortunate fact that most restaurants do not emphasize fresh foods and whole grains on the menus. Packing your lunch may help you get back to the basics of your diet and promote weight loss, especially if you are starting your meal with a nice salad or piece of fruit.

FACT

Whole foods are wonderful for your nutritional needs if they are prepared correctly, but they can easily become junk food. For example, a plain baked potato is a wonderful thing. High in fiber, low in calories, and filling, a potato is a great choice for a nutritious food. However, cover it in butter, fry it, and top it with cheese and bacon and this perfectly nutritious food becomes a bad idea.

Is Your Goal Weight Realistic?

So you've hit a plateau and you can't make the scale budge, no matter what you do. You've talked to your doctor, but the doctor seems unconcerned about the issue. Have you hit a plateau because your idea of your goal weight and that of your physician are not the same?

If your goal weight is unrealistically low, you may experience frustration and feel defeated, even if you have made tremendous progress. Your surgeon will take into account your starting weight, your body type, your age, and many other factors when determining a healthy goal weight for you. While you may dream of being rail-thin, that may not be a healthy or realistic goal for you. In fact, for many patients, a size 14 is a perfectly respectable goal and means a tremendous improvement in overall health benefits.

A goal weight is just that, a goal. That doesn't mean it is set in stone. You may find that the amount of exercise and calorie restrictions necessary to reach or maintain the targeted weight is unrealistic, or are so restrictive that you don't feel you can maintain the effort. If you are feeling that this is the case, talk to your surgeon. You may find that you are in agreement, or you may find that some simple changes in your plan can result in meeting your goal.

Don't Give Up!!

Perseverance is key when trying to lose weight, whether you have had surgery or not. Try to think of it as a marathon, not a sprint. The changes you are making in both your diet and your exercise habits are meant to be life-long, not a way to get to your goal so you can revert to your old habits.

As you get closer to reaching your goals, your weight loss will inevitably slow down. You may find yourself measuring your loss in ounces instead of pounds each week, but those ounces do add up. It may take more time than you would prefer, but a loss of a quarter or half of a pound each week will still mean that you are steadily losing weight and getting to where you want to be.

One Meal a Week

Plan for indulgences so you don't ruin all of your efforts with one overly large meal. It is an unfortunate truth that a week of effort, closely following your diet to the letter and exercising daily, can be erased with one bad meal. This is especially true as you get closer to your goal weight and are losing smaller amounts of weight each week.

If you do plan to indulge, the key is not to deny yourself all treats and special foods, but to compensate for them with diet and exercise. If you know you will be having more calories than usual on Saturday, you may want to shave 100 calories from your diet Monday through Friday. You can also increase your exercise for the week.

In addition to "banking" some calories, you may also want to consider having a healthy, low-calorie, and filling snack prior to having your "indulgence." This way you will be less likely to overeat, but you can still enjoy a treat.

In the end, it is important to remember that each and every calorie does add up, not just on a daily basis, but over time as well. That fact can also work in your favor, allowing you to plan well in advance for holidays, parties, and even a craving for a food you no longer eat on a regular basis.

Adjusting Your Exercise Routine

Exercise will be the foundation of your weight loss success. It will help you reach your goals, both with pounds lost and improving your overall health. Most importantly, exercise will help you maintain that loss over time.

If you are experiencing a plateau, you may need to increase the amount you exercise in order to continue losing weight. You can increase exercise in one or more ways: by increasing the length of your exercise sessions, the intensity of those sessions, or the frequency.

Increasing Intensity

Increasing the intensity at which you work out just means working out harder. If you are currently walking a mile in twenty minutes, it may be time to start trying to walk the same distance in fifteen or eighteen minutes. If you are able to walk at a brisk pace, you may want to consider adding hand weights, or increasing your pace to a slow jog.

You can also increase your intensity in short bursts, called interval training. For example, if you are currently walking a mile in twenty minutes, you would add a few minutes of walking at a fifteen-minute pace, then return to your twenty-minute pace. You will burn more calories, and you will also improve your stamina.

ALERT

If you are using a treadmill for your workout, it can be very easy to increase the intensity at which you work out. Just increase the incline, which approximates walking up a hill or a slight grade. You can walk the same speed but get a much more intense workout simply by making this small change.

Increasing the Number of Workouts

Increasing the number of workouts you do per week is a fantastic way to speed your weight loss. It can be as simple as adding a fifteen-minute walk to your after-dinner routine, or you can add a full-length gym workout to your day. Exercise does add up. If you are able to work out for half an hour, but an hour is too exhausting, consider a thirty-minute workout twice a day. Your stamina will improve and you will be doing an hour at a time before you know it.

Increasing the Length of Workouts

For maximum results, plan on working out for an hour, six days per week. If that isn't realistic, start with shorter workouts and increase the duration of your exercise a minute or two each week until you are able to consistently work out for an hour. If you are trying to increase the length of time you spend working out, but you are struggling to add time without feeling exhausted, consider adding 10 percent every two weeks. So if you are currently working out thirty minutes a day, add three minutes (10 percent) over the course of the next two weeks. Over time, you will reach your hour goal, but you won't feel like you are killing yourself to get there.

If your schedule is a big factor, try adding in mini workouts wherever you can. Mini workouts are barely a workout at all, but over time, the effort adds up.

EXAMPLES OF MINI WORKOUTS:

- Taking a flight or two of stairs instead of the elevator
- Parking your car at the far end of the parking lot instead of looking for the closest spot
- Taking your dog for a five-minute walk
- Turning up the radio and dancing around the house for five minutes
- Doing leg lifts while watching TV

Adding New Activities to Your Workout

If you are bored with your workout, tired of getting on the same treadmill every day, or doing the same exercise routine, it may be time to add some variety to your program. A wide variety of exercise does more than prevent your workout from becoming stale, it also helps exercise a wide variety of muscle groups and will provide better all-over toning.

You should also add weight training to your regime. You don't need to use barbells to get a good weight training workout. You can use weight machines if you have a gym membership, but you can also use resistance bands and techniques like Pilates to build muscle. Not only does toned muscle have an attractive appearance, it also will improve your metabolism.

Looking for Other Causes

In most cases, adjusting your diet, or increasing the amount of exercise you are doing will get your weight loss on track after a plateau. However, in a small minority of cases, there are other factors at work, making weight loss more difficult.

Hypothyroidism

Hypothyroidism is a disorder where the thyroid gland produces too little or no thyroid hormone. It can lead to weight gain along with fatigue that is not relieved by adequate sleep. While hypothyroidism can be easily treated with prescription medication, it may be overlooked as a cause of weight gain or a failure to lose weight.

FACT

Symptoms of hypothyroidism include coarse and/or dry hair, dry skin, hair loss, depression, constipation, irritability, decreased sex drive, and sensitivity to cold.

Prescription Medications

Some prescription medications can make it difficult to lose weight and can even cause weight gain. Many drugs can cause weight gain, including prescription medications for high blood pressure, depression, heartburn, diabetes, and more. If you are taking a prescription medication, be sure to review the side effects with your pharmacist or physician.

Chronic Stress

Chronic stress can make it difficult to lose weight in many ways. Stress is associated with difficulty sleeping, hormone changes, and altered blood sugar levels, which can all hinder weight loss. Stress can also cause emotional issues that lead to overeating and cravings for junk food and processed foods.

If your stress level is out of control, you may want to consider adding stress-relieving exercise to your plan, such as yoga or tai chi. While exercise may not remove stress from your life, it may make it easier to cope with stress and help get your weight loss back on track.

Water Retention

If you are consuming too much salt, or if you are approaching your menstrual period, you may be retaining water. Swollen fingers and ankles are usually the first indication that you are holding more water than usual, which can lead to an artificially increased body weight.

Oddly enough, the best treatment for mild water retention is to drink more water! Dehydration will cause your body to hold on to more water, while drinking adequate water will trigger your body to release excess stored water.

Scale Versus Measuring Tape

It is possible that you are continuing to lose inches and get healthier but you've added muscle mass, which means the scale isn't necessarily showing the improvement in your body. If you are exercising and doing weight-training or muscle-toning exercise, consider using a measuring tape as your measure of success instead of the scale.

CHAPTER 13

Long-Term Success

Getting to your goal weight is only the beginning of the journey. Maintaining your weight loss and your good health is a lifelong process that doesn't stop when the pounds are gone. You might decide to have plastic surgery to continue to improve your appearance, or you may find that you need ongoing support to keep your weight in a healthy range.

Sticking with the Program

The single most important thing you can do to have great results long term is to stick with the program your surgeon prescribes. That means eating the right foods in the right amounts, exercising regularly, and taking care of your emotional health.

Sticking with it also means getting back on track after a bad day, a bad weekend, or even a bad week. It means going to the gym to make up for overindulging at dinner the night before, or working out a few extra times a week to compensate for a treat you are planning. Being accountable to yourself for every morsel you eat will make all the difference in your long-term weight maintenance.

If you have reached your goal weight, or if you've lost a significant amount of weight, you've learned a great deal about how to effectively lose weight, and you've also learned to cope with all of the changes that weight loss surgery brings. Reaching your goal doesn't mean you no longer need those skills; in fact, you will need them more than ever, making sure your hard work pays off for the future.

Keep Your Doctor's Appointments

A big part of long-term weight maintenance, as well as the maintenance of your good health, is keeping your appointments with your doctors. You may think that these visits are just about your weight, and perhaps not very important, but they serve a far greater purpose. Your surgeon and your primary physician will help make sure that you are not suffering from any ill effects brought on by surgery, such as vitamin and mineral deficiencies, malnutrition, osteoporosis, a hernia at your surgical site, or other potential complications post–weight loss surgery. They can also detect any conditions that could hinder your long-term results, such as hypothyroidism.

These visits also serve another purpose: They encourage you to follow your diet plan, as every one of these visits will include hopping on the scale. If you are not someone who likes using the scale to measure your progress, these checkups will be an opportunity to weigh in without feeling as though you are a slave to your bathroom scale.

Medical Conditions

Over the course of your weight loss journey, you may be pleasantly surprised by how much your medical conditions improve. Patients with type 2 diabetes, high blood pressure, and even sleep apnea often experience a dramatic improvement or full reversal of their problems as they lose weight. These conditions should continue to be closely monitored, as any medication you are taking may need to be adjusted frequently, or even discontinued.

Just because you are now thin doesn't mean you can quit taking your medication. While many people do benefit from losing weight and are able to completely quit taking their prescription medications, don't assume you are one of them. Your doctor may need to run tests to determine if your medication can be changed, decreased, or discontinued, but don't assume you can stop until you are told to do so.

Evaluating Your Habits

Weight loss surgery can do amazing things, and can bring about great changes in your habits. Creating healthy new habits and eliminating unhealthy or harmful habits is a big part of the weight loss process, but keeping in touch with your new habits is very important. For example, immediately after your surgery you may weigh or measure every bit of food you eat. Then, when you become confident in your ability to judge portion sizes, you no longer feel the need to measure. Over time, your portions can slowly become larger and larger, until you are no longer following your plan. To combat slipping into old habits, old portion sizes, and other problems, plan on "checking in" on a regular basis.

Once a month, or as often as necessary, plan on measuring your food, just to make sure your portions haven't grown. Make sure that walk you take, which you do faster and faster over time, still lasts an hour. You can even have a "maintenance" visit with your support group or therapist, if you've gotten away from going regularly.

Food Diary

Your food diary may be more important when you are maintaining your weight than at any other time. You've adjusted to the foods you can and cannot eat, your pouch (if you had a restrictive surgery) can accommodate a more "normal" sized meal, which means this is also the time when you can slip back into eating junk foods, sweets, and other nutritionally deficient foods.

A food diary, even if you don't use it every day, can be a very useful tool when you are trying to make sure that you aren't consuming more calories than you should. It can also help you determine if specific foods are causing an upset stomach. Or if you are gaining weight, it can help you and your doctor find a cause.

The Scale

The scale is both a great tool and a cause of stress and anger. If you are motivated by the scale, by all means use it as frequently as you like. Many people need to find alternative ways to measure their progress, such as trying on the same pair of jeans each week to see how they fit, taking their measurements, or even using fat calipers to determine their percentage of body fat.

Rather than feeling obligated to use a scale, decide what method of measuring your current body weight works best for you, and use it regularly.

FACT

Consider choosing a day where you weigh yourself, whether it is once a week or once a month, and not deviating from that plan. You can also get rid of your scale altogether and stop into your doctor's office when you feel the need to weigh in. You don't need to have an appointment to use the scale, and it will keep you from torturing yourself with the scale on a daily basis.

Exercise Diary

An exercise diary, like a food diary, can help keep you honest when it comes to how much exercise you are doing and at what intensity. This way, if you notice a weight gain, you can determine if you've been consuming more calories, exercising less, or if something else could be contributing to the issue.

Keeping track of your exercise in a diary is a good idea for another reason: You may find that one exercise leads to more weight loss than a different exercise. If you track your exercise and your weight loss, you might spot a trend that helps you decide which types of exercises lead to improved weight loss, versus those that don't make much of an impact.

The diary isn't just about making sure you maintain your weight, it can be a fantastic way to measure your progress and see how far you've come. Imagine going from only being able to walk for a few minutes at a time to being able to walk or run for long distances. This kind of progress should be noted and rewarded as you meet milestone goals.

Enjoying Your Success

You've made it! You've learned a new way to eat, you've added exercise to your life, and you've learned tools and tricks for dealing with problems that arise without turning to food.

Take the time to really think about all you've accomplished, and how much work you've done to reach this point. You've spent countless hours working out, reading food labels, and cooking meals at home. It is time to truly celebrate all that you've done. While having a party and celebrating with too much food isn't appropriate, finding ways to acknowledge your triumph over excess weight shouldn't be too difficult! Start with all of the things about which you always said, "I'd love to do that, maybe when I'm thin." Maybe you've been putting off a vacation to a location where you would wear a bathing suit, or visiting somewhere that would require a great deal of walking. You no longer have a good reason not to do either of those things!

New Body

Not only do you look better, you should be feeling much better too! Aches and pains should be dramatically better, you should have more energy, and you may even be off prescription medications. Your body is as happy about the changes you've made as you are!

It may take time to truly appreciate your new body. You may find it hard to believe that you are truly at your goal weight, or you may be more focused on the imperfections that you see rather than the improvements. Appreciate your newly found good health, and be thankful that you have been able to stick to your goals.

The people around you surely have noticed that you have accomplished some amazing things. You are probably receiving all sorts of positive comments about your appearance from many different people. Enjoy this time and all the new changes that you have earned.

New Clothes

One of the things that many weight loss surgery patients have in common is the joy they feel when shopping for clothing. No longer being limited to a few stores or a small section of a store can be exhilarating, and you may find that you are able to wear things that you never dreamed you could.

It may not be easy to shop at first, especially if you are accustomed to wearing things that are oversized or even shapeless. You might need to bring a friend along as a second opinion, as what was flattering in the past may not be the best choice now. Just remember to enjoy the first time you drop a size and the first time you need to go shopping because absolutely everything is too big. These are the moments that you have been hoping for, so try not to view shopping for new clothing as a chore. Enjoy your newfound ability to shop wherever you please, and don't hesitate to use clothing as a reward for consistently eating well and working out.

New Outlook on Life

You may find that you have a different outlook on life, a more upbeat way of approaching your day, after losing weight. For many, weight loss means more energy, less pain, less medication, and less stress. With all of those positive changes, it is hard not to see the world differently, to take more pleasure in your life.

While life won't be perfect because of weight loss, it can dramatically improve when your feet and back no longer ache, when you wake up each morning ready to bounce out of bed, and when you like what you see in the mirror. It is hard not to have a drastic improvement in your self esteem when you've lost weight, and that will certainly have an effect on how you perceive and are perceived in your day-to-day life.

Plastic Surgery

Plastic surgery may be necessary or desirable after losing a large amount of weight. Rapid and extensive weight loss can lead to excess skin. A loss of elasticity is common after weight loss, so even as weight is lost, the skin doesn't necessarily shrink to fit the body. You may also find that, even at your goal weight, you desire a more contoured appearance than exercise and weight loss can provide.

QUESTION

After weight loss surgery, plastic surgery isn't a big deal, is it?
Plastic surgery is as serious as any other surgery you might need, including weight loss surgery. All surgeries have risks, up to and including the risk of death! Don't believe for a moment that plastic surgery isn't serious just because you won't need to stay in a hospital overnight once it is over.

Plastic surgery is a very personal decision. Some are thrilled to be much thinner and feel no need for any additional "improvements," while others want to look as good as possible and feel that surgery is a natural step after significant weight loss. Like weight loss surgery, plastic surgery has risks and should not be taken lightly. While you are probably a far better surgical candidate after losing weight, every surgery has the possibility of complications.

Like your weight loss surgery, it is essential to be diligent in selecting a surgeon who is board certified in plastic surgery and has regularly performed the surgery you desire. The skill of the surgeon will be the most important decision you make in terms of the final result.

Plastic surgery can be very expensive, and it is rarely covered by insurance. In some cases, where it is deemed medically necessary, insurance may pay for surgery expenses. Those situations typically include removing excess skin when it is a source of chronic skin irritation or infection.

When to Have Plastic Surgery

Plastic surgery can be very beneficial in helping you achieve the body that you desire. In many cases, dramatic weight loss doesn't lead to the beautiful body that you may have expected; it can result in extra skin that hangs from your body, breasts that look deflated, and even skin folds that cause chronic skin irritation.

If you decide that plastic surgery is for you, it is important that you wait for at least a year after you reach your goal weight. This is for several reasons. You will have a better overall outcome from your surgery if your weight is no longer fluctuating. It is possible that you may not feel the need for surgery after your skin has had time to adjust to your new body, and most importantly, a year will give you the time you need to get used to your new appearance and decide what is right for you long term.

For some, plastic surgery is more need than desire. Skin folds can be irritated and red, due to yeast and other skin problems. The skin under the breasts, like other skin folds, can be raw and harbor moisture or a fungal infection. For these problems, removing excess skin can treat the problem permanently.

ALERT

Will you feel better once you've had plastic surgery, or will you just find something else that needs to be done, in order to improve your appearance? Be sure that surgery is what you want and that the improvement will truly be an improvement to your life. Take the time to really think about whether your dissatisfaction with your appearance will be resolved with surgery, or if what you feel is truly on the inside rather than the outside.

When to Wait for Plastic Surgery

If you are considering plastic surgery, you may consider waiting if any of the following apply to you:

- Your weight is not stable.
- You have not been at your goal weight for a full year.
- You are planning to become pregnant.
- You are having difficulty maintaining a healthy minimum weight.
- You are having difficulty staying at your goal weight (it can be difficult to exercise after surgery).
- You have another health condition that makes surgery risky.

When Surgery Isn't Successful

In rare cases, weight loss surgery is not successful, either in the short term or the long term. For others, after significant initial weight loss, the pounds creep back on, leading to significant weight gain. Unfortunately, it is possible to have weight loss surgery and be the same starting weight a few years later.

Determining the nature of why surgery was not successful is the most important thing you can do, as it will determine what is done in the future to correct the problem. If it is a behavioral issue, such as overeating or not exercising, your surgeon may recommend further therapy or visits with a nutritionist. If there was a problem with the procedure itself, tests may be performed to determine the exact nature of the problem. Your surgeon may suggest a surgical revision or another less invasive solution.

If the surgery was performed correctly and you have followed your surgeon's instructions, testing may be necessary to determine why it was not as successful as was expected.

Evaluating Why It Didn't Work

Before you decide what to do, you need to determine why your weight loss surgery did not work. Did you experience complications that undermined your results? Did you have difficulty adhering to the dietary restrictions that your surgeon recommended? Did you have a medical problem that interfered with your ability to lose weight, such as hypothyroidism? Did you adhere to the post–weight loss surgery diet but chose not to exercise? Perhaps you made the necessary changes long enough to lose weight, or even long enough to achieve your goal weight, but then slipped back into your old habits.

Your surgeon may also have insight into why your surgery did not provide the expected results. If there was a problem with the surgical procedure itself, a "redo," or new surgery to fix the problem, may be necessary. Generally speaking, problems with the actual surgical procedure or the restructured anatomy are not as common as patients who do not make the necessary changes that allow them to lose weight.

Revision

A revision is a surgical procedure that is done to fix a problem with the original surgery. For example, if the stomach pouch initially left by the surgeon is too large or has stretched too much, a revision procedure might be done to decrease the size.

If your surgery has not been successful, or your surgeon has concerns about the function of your digestive system after the procedure, a revision may be suggested.

Reversal

A reversal surgery is done to return the anatomy of the body to the condition it was prior to surgery, or as close as possible. A reversal of a gastric bypass would reroute the intestine so that digested food passed through the entire intestine, rather than bypassing a large portion of it.

While the need for a reversal is rare, it is most often performed when the patient has lost too much weight, or cannot stop losing weight. While it may sound like a dream come true to lose too much weight, for these patients the inability to absorb enough calories leads to serious complications and can be life threatening.

Band Erosion

Gastric banding procedures encircle the stomach with an adjustable band. This band can, over time, cause erosion of the stomach where it touches the band. In most cases, the band must be removed to prevent further damage to the stomach and to allow the area to heal.

CHAPTER 14

Liquid and Soft-Food Recipes

Pancakes

Pancakes are filling, but they are also soft enough to eat when your stomach cannot tolerate crisp foods or foods that are more difficult to digest.

INGREDIENTS | YIELDS 3 PORTIONS OF 2 PANCAKES EACH

1½ cups whole wheat flour

¼ teaspoon salt

3 tablespoons baking powder

1 tablespoon vegetable oil

1¾ cups soy milk or fat-free milk

Whole Wheat Flour

Whole wheat flour has much more nutritional value than white flour. The same is true of whole wheat bread versus white bread. Substitute whole-grain or whole wheat products for more refined products wherever you can to increase the vitamins and minerals in your diet.

1. Combine and sift flour, salt, and baking powder.

2. In a medium bowl, combine oil and milk and whip for 1 minute until frothy.

3. Combine wet and dry mixes until well blended.

4. Spray nonstick skillet with cooking spray and place over medium heat. Ladle batter onto skillet with a 2-ounce ladle (approximately 4 inches in diameter).

5. Wait until you see bubbles rise and begin popping, approximately 2–3 minutes, then flip once and cook an additional 2–3 minutes or until lightly browned and serve.

PER SERVING: Calories: 300 | Fat: 6g | Protein: 13g | Sodium: 1740mg | Fiber: 7g | Carbohydrates: 55g

Chunky Apple Sauce Muffins

These muffins are packed with flavor, but don't have the fat and calories that most commercially produced muffins are hiding.

INGREDIENTS | YIELDS 12 MUFFINS

2 cups whole wheat flour

2 teaspoons baking powder

1 teaspoon arrow root powder

½ teaspoon allspice

2 teaspoons cinnamon

¼ teaspoon cloves

¼ teaspoon ginger powder

½ cup sorghum

½ cup unsweetened apple sauce

2 apples, peeled and sliced

½ cup water

½ teaspoon vanilla

1. Preheat oven to 400°F.

2. Mix flour, baking powder, arrow root powder, allspice, cinnamon, cloves, and ginger powder.

3. In a separate bowl, mix sorghum, apple sauce, apples, water, and vanilla.

4. Combine both mixes, spray muffin pans with nonstick spray, and fill halfway with batter.

5. Bake for 25 minutes, cool, and serve.

PER MUFFIN: Calories: 110 | Fat: 0.5g | Protein: 4g | Sodium: 0mg | Fiber: 4g | Carbohydrates: 25g

Replacing Fat with Applesauce

If you have a cake or brownie recipe that calls for added oil, consider substituting applesauce. The applesauce provides sweetness and moisture for your recipe without the added fat and calories of oil.

Super Scramble

A low-fat, high-protein version of a breakfast staple.

INGREDIENTS | SERVES 1

Nonstick cooking spray

2 white mushrooms, sliced

2 teaspoons red bell peppers, diced

½ cup egg whites

¼ cup firm tofu

3 tablespoons low-fat Cheddar cheese

1. Heat nonstick pan over medium heat. Spray with nonstick cooking spray and add mushrooms and peppers. Cook until tender, about 2–3 minutes.

2. Add eggs and tofu. Scramble eggs over low heat with wooden spoon until done, approximately 3–4 minutes.

3. Add cheese and serve.

PER SERVING: Calories: 190 | Fat: 7g | Protein: 28g | Sodium: 340mg | Fiber: 1g | Carbohydrates: 5g

Zucchini-Onion Quiche

A quiche is a great high-protein way to start the day, but the crust can be high in fat. This quiche uses rice for the crust, for a guilt-free breakfast or brunch.

INGREDIENTS | YIELDS 1 (9-INCH) QUICHE; SERVING SIZE 9 (1-INCH) PIECES

1 cup long grain rice, cooked

1 cup shredded Swiss cheese (fat free or low fat)

3 egg whites, divided use

1 medium onion, chopped

1 carrot, peeled and grated

1 zucchini, grated

1 cup low-sodium chicken broth

1 teaspoon crumbled basil

1 cup skim milk

1. Preheat oven to 425°F. Spray pan with nonstick spray.

2. Mix rice, 2 tablespoons of cheese, and 1 egg white in a bowl. Moisten hands then press mixture into pan in the shape of a pie crust. Place in oven and bake for 5 minutes.

3. Combine onion, carrot, zucchini, chicken broth, and basil in a sauté pan. Cook over medium heat until veggies are softened, but still crisp. Remove from heat.

4. Combine cooked ingredients with skim milk, cheese, and remaining egg whites; pour into prebaked shell. Reduce oven to 350°F and bake for 20–25 minutes.

PER SERVING: Calories: 190 | Fat: 1g | Protein: 7g | Sodium: 75mg | Fiber: <1g | Carbohydrates: 10g

Super-Nutritious Smoothie

This smoothie has an amazing combination of ingredients designed to provide abundant protein, vitamins, and minerals in a quick and easy drink.

INGREDIENTS | SERVES 4

1 ripe banana, peeled

½ apple, peeled and cored

1 kiwi, peeled

½ cup frozen mixed berries

1 cup orange juice

½ cup soy milk (or rice milk, fat-free milk, or almond milk)

½ cup fat-free yogurt (flavored if preferred)

½ cup tofu

3 tablespoons peanut butter

1. Combine all ingredients in blender. Blend until smooth.

2. Use immediately or refrigerate for use the next day.

PER SERVING: Calories: 210 | Fat: 8g | Protein: 9g | Sodium: 40mg | Fiber: 3g | Carbohydrates: 27g

Kiwi Mango Smoothie

This smoothie is a cool and refreshing way to start the day. It is also a soft but flavorful meal that can be eaten while you are recovering from surgery and can only eat liquids and soft foods.

INGREDIENTS | YIELDS 1½ CUPS; SERVES 2

1 kiwi fruit, peeled

⅓ cup mango (you can use canned, but fresh is better)

⅓ cup mango juice or white grape juice

⅓ cup plain, fat-free yogurt

1 teaspoon flaxseeds

4 ice cubes

1 mint sprig to garnish, optional

1. Cut kiwi and mango into chunks.

2. Combine all ingredients except mint in blender, blend until smooth.

3. Pour into glass. If desired, garnish with mint.

PER SERVING: Calories: 100 | Fat: 1g | Protein: 3g | Sodium: 35mg | Fiber: 2g | Carbohydrates: 200g

Flaxseed

Adding flaxseed to a smoothie is a great way to increase the amount of protein and fiber in your drink.

Green Tea Smoothie

If you need a pick-me-up in the morning, or you are just bored with all of the soft foods
\that you are permitted to eat, this smoothie is a great alternative!

INGREDIENTS | SERVES 2

2 cups fat-free milk
¼ cup unsweetened instant tea granules (preferably green)
¼ cup nonfat vanilla yogurt
¼ teaspoon cinnamon
¼ teaspoon ginger
¼ teaspoon cardamom
1 cup ice cubes
1 teaspoon honey

Combine ingredients in a blender, blend until smooth.

PER SERVING: Calories: 218 | Fat: 0g | Protein: 17g | Sodium: 170mg | Fiber: 2g | Carbohydrates: 38g

Protein Power Smoothie

This smoothie provides the protein you need with the flavor you want.
Adding protein powder helps boost your protein intake without adding too many calories.

INGREDIENTS | SERVES 2

1 scoop protein powder (flavored if you prefer)
½ cup low-fat or fat-free cottage cheese
¼ cup milk (soy, rice, or regular)
1 cup water
1 cup ice cubes
½ cup pineapple
½ cup mango

Combine all ingredients in blender. Blend until smooth.

PER SERVING: Calories: 150 | Fat: 0.5g | Protein: 21g | Sodium: 350mg | Fiber: 2g | Carbohydrates: 15g

Cottage Cheese

Cottage cheese is a great way to replace higher-fat cheese in recipes or add a creamy texture to smoothies.

Papaya Banana Smoothie

For a cool and refreshing breakfast, try this smoothie.
Loaded with protein and fiber, this drink is a filling way to start the day.

INGREDIENTS | SERVES 2

1 cup fat-free milk

¼ cup fat-free vanilla yogurt

1 small ripe banana, peeled

½ large papaya

1 cup ice

Combine all ingredients in blender. Blend until smooth, serve immediately.

PER SERVING: Calories: 150 | Fat: 0g | Protein: 7g | Sodium: 90mg | Fiber: 3g | Carbohydrates: 33g

Protein Power!

If you are struggling to get more protein into your diet, add protein powder to your smoothie. You can even find protein powders in flavors like vanilla, a perfect compliment to the vanilla yogurt in this recipe.

Wheat Germ Smoothie

Wheat germ adds both fiber and protein to your diet. If you are struggling to get enough protein each day, wheat germ may be the solution you need.

INGREDIENTS | YIELDS 3 CUPS; SERVING SIZE 1 CUP

1 ripe medium banana

1 cup vanilla low-fat or nonfat yogurt

¼ cup fresh orange juice

¼ cup wheat germ

1 cup ice

1 cup sliced fresh peaches

1. Place all ingredients except ice in blender and blend until smooth.

2. Add ice and blend until smooth. Serve immediately.

PER SERVING: Calories: 180 | Fat: 1.5g | Protein: 8g | Sodium: 55mg | Fiber: 4g | Carbohydrates: 36g

Avocado Tofu Smoothie

Avocado and tofu are both high in vitamins and minerals. Adding both to your breakfast is a great way to pack extra nutrients into your day. Avocado can also help boost your good cholesterol.

INGREDIENTS | SERVES 2

½ avocado, peeled

Juice of 1 lime

1 cup low-fat coconut milk or soy milk, chilled

½ cup silken tofu

½ medium cucumber, peeled and seeded

Combine all ingredients in blender. Blend until smooth.

PER SERVING: Calories: 170 | Fat: 10g | Protein: 6g | Sodium: 55mg | Fiber: 4g | Carbohydrates: 16g

Coconut Milk

Refrigerating coconut milk, even low-fat coconut milk, will cause the fat to rise to the top, where it can be easily removed. Keep the flavor of the coconut milk, but discard the fat that you don't need.

Peaches and Cream Smoothie

This smoothie is creamy and rich, without the added fat and calories of whipped cream or full-fat milk. It is a great way to replace creamy drinks that are diet disasters.

INGREDIENTS | SERVES 2

1 cup frozen peaches

1 tablespoon honey

⅓ cup pasteurized egg whites

½ cup fat-free milk

½ cup low-fat vanilla yogurt

Combine all ingredients in blender. Blend until smooth and frothy.

PER SERVING: Calories: 160 | Fat: 1g | Protein: 10g | Sodium: 140mg | Fiber: 1g | Carbohydrates: 29g

Pasteurized Egg Whites

Pasteurized egg whites can help make breakfast quick and easy. If you like to add protein to your smoothies, or if you like egg white omelets or scrambled eggs, these egg whites come in a carton so you don't need to crack or separate eggs.

Very Berry Smoothie

This smoothie is a great addition to any brunch or breakfast.
Sized to share, this smoothie is low in calories for you, but tasty enough for the rest of the family.

INGREDIENTS | SERVES 4

1 cup frozen strawberries
1 cup frozen blackberries
1 cup frozen peaches
1 cup raspberry sorbet (low-fat or sugar-free if possible)
1 cup orange juice

Combine all ingredients in a blender. Blend until smooth. Serve immediately.

PER SERVING: Calories: 140 | Fat: 0g | Protein: 1g | Sodium: 0mg | Fiber: 4g | Carbohydrates: 35g

Change It Up!

Try pomegranate or cherry juice for tartness, apple juice for sweetness, or grape juice for both. Just avoid juices where sugar was added, as you don't need the added sugar or calories, just the natural juice.

Tofu Smoothie

Tofu is a great way to add protein without adding fat or too many calories.
It will also give your smoothies a creamy texture without adding dairy.

INGREDIENTS | SERVES 2

1 cup frozen raspberries
1 cup crushed pineapple, with juice
½ cup coconut milk
2 tablespoons honey
½ cup silken tofu

Combine all ingredients in blender. Blend until smooth.

PER SERVING: Calories: 320 | Fat: 14g | Protein: 7g | Sodium: 30mg | Fiber: 6g | Carbohydrates: 47g

Tofu and Vitamins

Tofu is an excellent source of B vitamins. If you are struggling to get enough B vitamins in your diet, consider adding tofu to your breakfast smoothies and stir fries, or even try grilling tofu.

Orange Maple Smoothie

*The refreshing flavor of orange is combined with the sweet flavor
of maple syrup for a sweet breakfast treat.*

INGREDIENTS | SERVES 4

1 pint soy milk or fat-free milk

1 cup orange juice

½ cup maple syrup

1 large ripe banana, peeled

½ teaspoon cinnamon

1 cup ice

Combine ingredients in blender. Blend until smooth.
Serve immediately.

PER SERVING: Calories: 210 | Fat: 0g | Protein: 5g |
Sodium: 70mg | Fiber: 1g | Carbohydrates: 48g

Soy Milk

Soy milk is available in multiple flavors,
including vanilla and chocolate. Add flavor
to your smoothies, cereal, and other foods
you use milk with by substituting flavored
soy milk.

Banana Cherry Smoothie

*Milk, protein powder, and vanilla yogurt give this drink a high protein content.
Start your day with a blast of protein.*

INGREDIENTS | SERVES 2

1 banana, chunked and frozen

2 cups frozen cherries

1 cup fat-free milk

½ cup fat-free vanilla yogurt

½ cup pomegranate juice or orange
juice

1 tablespoon honey

2 tablespoons protein powder

Combine all ingredients in blender, blend until
smooth.

PER SERVING: Calories: 350 | Fat: 0.5g | Protein: 22g |
Sodium: 240mg | Fiber: 5g | Carbohydrates: 69g

Pomegranate and Cranberry Soda

If you are looking for a change from water but you don't want to add empty calories to your diet, try this sparkling and fruity alternative.

INGREDIENTS | YIELDS 1 PITCHER; SERVING SIZE 1 CUP

3 cups chilled unsweetened cranberry juice

¾ cup chilled pomegranate juice

⅓ cup fresh lime juice

6 packets of no-calorie sweetener

3 cups chilled club soda

1. In large pitcher, combine juices then slowly stir in sweetener until dissolved.

2. Add club soda and mix to combine. Pour into glasses and serve.

PER SERVING: Calories: 140 | Fat: 0g | Protein: 1g | Sodium: 30mg | Fiber: 0g | Carbohydrates: 39g

Apple Rice Milk Smoothie

Apple juice and fresh apples combine to give this smoothie a tart and tangy flavor. If you are having trouble getting fresh fruit into your diet, this smoothie will do the trick.

INGREDIENTS | SERVES 2

1 cup banana chunks, frozen

¾ cup rice milk, chilled

½ Granny Smith apple, cored and chunked

¼ cup apple juice, chilled

2 fresh peppermint leaves

1. Combine all ingredients except the peppermint in blender and blend until smooth.

2. Garnish with fresh peppermint leaves, serve immediately.

PER SERVING: Calories: 150 | Fat: 1g | Protein: 2g | Sodium: 35mg | Fiber: 3g | Carbohydrates: 36g

Apple Peels

If you are trying to get more fiber into your diet, wash your fruit and vegetables thoroughly but leave the peels on. This will increase the vitamin and mineral content in your diet too.

Peach Rice Milk Smoothie

*Using frozen bananas and peaches makes this smoothie thick and creamy,
a real treat that adds 2 servings of fruit to your day.*

INGREDIENTS | SERVES 2

1 banana, cut into chunks and frozen

1 cup rice milk, chilled

1 cup frozen peaches

1 tablespoon orange juice

Combine ingredients in blender, blend until smooth.
Serve immediately.

PER SERVING: Calories: 160 | Fat: 1.5g | Protein: 3g |
Sodium: 45mg | Fiber: 4g | Carbohydrates: 37g

Frozen Fruit

If you have trouble using fruit before it
goes bad, consider buying frozen fruit from
your supermarket. You can use as much or
as little as you need without having it go
bad in your refrigerator and it also helps
keep your smoothie cold while you drink it.

High-Protein Breakfast Smoothie

*This smoothie packs a protein punch that is hard to beat.
You can even save some in the refrigerator for the next day.*

**INGREDIENTS | YIELDS 3 CUPS; SERVING
SIZE 1 CUP**

1 banana

½ apple, peeled

1 kiwi, peeled

½ cup frozen mixed berries

1 cup orange juice

½ cup soy milk

½ cup nonfat plain yogurt

½ cup tofu

3 tablespoons natural peanut butter

2 tablespoons flaxseed oil

1. In a blender, combine banana, apple, kiwi, mixed
   berries, and orange juice. Blend until smooth.

2. Add soy milk, yogurt, tofu, peanut butter, and flaxseed
   oil, and blend again until smooth.

PER SERVING: Calories: 370 | Fat: 20g | Protein: 12g |
Sodium: 60mg | Fiber: 5g | Carbohydrates: 37g

Melon Smoothie Cooler

If you like melons, this smoothie is for you. Watermelon and cantaloupe combine with a hint of lime and cool yogurt to make a fat-free smoothie that tastes like summer.

INGREDIENTS | SERVES 4

1½ cups watermelon, peeled and seeded

1½ cups cantaloupe, peeled and seeded

Juice of 2 limes

1 cup fat-free vanilla yogurt

1 cup ice cubes

1. Combine ingredients in blender, blend until smooth.

2. If you desire to serve the smoothie on different days, omit the ice, chill, and serve over ice as desired.

PER SERVING: Calories: 100 | Fat: 0g | Protein: 4g | Sodium: 50mg | Fiber: < 1g | Carbohydrates: 22g

Melons

Melons are a great food for weight loss. High in fiber and low in calories, they are nutritious and full of flavor. Watermelon is a great snack because it has so few calories that you can eat enough to feel full without ruining your diet for the day.

CHAPTER 15

Marinades, Dressings, and Rubs

Lime Yogurt Marinade for Chicken

This flavorful marinade is given a unique twist with the tangy and tart taste of lime yogurt. Marinate your chicken in this for a low-fat and high-protein meal with all of the flavor of a high-fat dish.

INGREDIENTS | YIELDS 1 CUP

1 tablespoon lime juice

½ tablespoon red wine vinegar

1 garlic clove

1 teaspoon Dijon mustard

6 tablespoons plain nonfat yogurt

¼ teaspoon salt

Fresh ground black pepper, to taste

Combine lime juice, vinegar, clove, Dijon mustard, yogurt, salt, and pepper in a bowl. Mix thoroughly. Use immediately or refrigerate up to one week.

PER RECIPE: Calories: 50 | Fat: 0g | Protein: 4g | Sodium: 760mg | Fiber: 0g | Carbohydrates: 10g

Chicken Safety

Raw chicken can carry salmonella, but careful washing of your hands, counters, and cutting boards will make your kitchen much safer.

Asian Marinade

Low-sodium soy sauce gives this marinade great flavor without loading your diet down with unwanted salt.

INGREDIENTS | YIELDS 1¼ CUPS

½ cup fresh orange juice

3 tablespoons low-sodium soy sauce

¼ yellow onion, thinly sliced

1 clove garlic, smashed

¼ teaspoon sesame oil

½ teaspoon five-spice powder

1 inch fresh ginger root, peeled and chopped

¼ cup water

1 red Thai chili pepper, seeded

1. Combine all ingredients and mix to combine.

2. Store covered in refrigerator until ready to use.

PER RECIPE: Calories: 130 | Fat: 2g | Protein: 5g | Sodium: 1610mg | Fiber: 2g | Carbohydrates: 27g

Avocado Dressing

Tons of flavor with little to no fat and bright flavors.
This dressing also makes an excellent dip for fresh vegetables.

INGREDIENTS | YIELDS 1 CUP

1 ripe avocado, pitted and peeled
½ cup fat-free or low-fat buttermilk
Pinch of ground cayenne
Juice of 1 lime
½ teaspoon granulated garlic
3 tablespoons fresh cilantro, chopped
Salt and pepper, to taste
¼ teaspoon ground cumin
¼ cup fat-free sour cream

Place all ingredients in a food processor. Blend in short pulses until thick and smooth.

PER 2 TABLESPOONS: Calories: 60 | Fat: 4g | Protein: 2g | Sodium: 20mg | Fiber: 2g | Carbohydrates: 5g

BBQ Spiced Rub

Lip-smacking BBQ flavor to season chicken or pork with no added salt.

INGREDIENTS | YIELDS ½ CUP

1 teaspoon dry mustard
½ teaspoon cracked black pepper
½ teaspoon ground cumin
1 tablespoon brown sugar
1 tablespoon chili powder
1 teaspoon garlic powder
1 teaspoon onion powder
1 teaspoon dry thyme
1 teaspoon smoked paprika

Mix all ingredients to combine. Store in an airtight container until ready to use.

PER SERVING: Calories: 130 | Fat: 3g | Protein: 3g | Sodium: 90mg | Fiber: 5g | Carbohydrates: 25g

Buttermilk Marinade

Buttermilk gives this marinade a tangy zip like you would expect from southern fried chicken and other southern chicken recipes. Lots of flavor, but the low-fat buttermilk keeps it from being a diet disaster.

INGREDIENTS | YIELDS 1½ CUPS

1 cup low-fat buttermilk

¼ cup fat-free sour cream

¼ teaspoon cracked black pepper

2 teaspoons lemon juice

2 tablespoons dried chives

2 shallots, peeled and chopped

⅛ teaspoon cayenne

Combine all ingredients and mix thoroughly.

PER RECIPE: Calories: 220 | Fat: 3g | Protein: 13g | Sodium: 310mg | Fiber: < 1g | Carbohydrates: 36g

Buttermilk Enzymes

The enzymes in buttermilk work to tenderize meat when it is used as a marinade.

Chinese Five-Spice Rub

This intensely flavored rub replaces the flavor lost when fat is eliminated from your pork and chicken recipes.

INGREDIENTS | YIELDS 2.5 OUNCES (GOOD FOR ONE LARGE CHICKEN)

1½ tablespoons Chinese five-spice powder

2 tablespoons canola oil

2 drops sesame oil

1 tablespoon water

3 tablespoons ground dried Shiitake mushrooms

Combine all ingredients and store in airtight container until ready to use.

PER RECIPE: Calories: 430 | Fat: 32g | Protein: 9g | Sodium: 25mg | Fiber: 3g | Carbohydrates: 34g

Chinese Five-Spice Powder

Once found only in Asian food markets, five-spice powder has entered the mainstream and can now be found in most grocery stores with a large spice selection.

Citrus Marinade

Bright fruity flavors add zing to food without the fat and sodium in most commercially prepared marinades. Great on salmon and chicken!

INGREDIENTS | YIELDS 1 CUP

¼ cup fresh orange juice

½ ounce lemon juice

¼ cup frozen limeade (frozen drink mix)

Zest of 1 lime and 1 orange each

½ cup water

2 tablespoons canola oil

1 bay leaf

1 teaspoon dried tarragon

Mix all ingredients to combine and store in refrigerator until ready to use.

PER SERVING: Calories: 280 | Fat: 28g | Protein: 1g | Sodium: 0mg | Fiber: 0g | Carbohydrates: 9g

Super-Garlic Meat Rub

A rub for garlic lovers with lots of flavor and the heart-healthy aspects of garlic.

INGREDIENTS | YIELDS ½ CUP; SERVING SIZE 1 TABLESPOON PER 4 OUNCES OF MEAT

2 tablespoons minced garlic

2 tablespoons roasted garlic puree

1 tablespoon granulated garlic

1 tablespoon granulated onion

1 teaspoon cracked black pepper

2 tablespoons canola oil

2 tablespoons dried Italian seasoning

1 teaspoon red wine vinegar

¼ teaspoon kosher salt

Combine all ingredients and mix well. Store covered in refrigerator until ready to use.

PER TABLESPOON: Calories: 60 | Fat: 4.5g | Protein: 1g | Sodium: 120mg | Fiber: <1g | Carbohydrates: 4g

Hot and Spicy Marinade

Low in sodium and fat free, this is a great way to flavor protein and marinate fresh vegetables before roasting. This marinade also is a fantastic way to start baked chicken wings.

INGREDIENTS | YIELDS 1 CUP

½ cup Low Sodium Frank's Red Hot

¼ cup fresh orange juice

¼ cup water

1 teaspoon ground cumin

1 teaspoon light chili powder

1 teaspoon granulated garlic powder

Mix all ingredients to combine and store covered in refrigerator until ready to use.

PER SERVING: Calories: 120 | Fat: 1g | Protein: 2g | Sodium: 830mg | Fiber: 2g | Carbohydrates: 24g

Like It Hot?

If you love spicy food, take care not to overdo it immediately after surgery, especially in the first few months.

Italian Dressing

Lower in fat and sugar than store-bought dressing, this flavorful dressing does double duty as a marinade.

INGREDIENTS | YIELDS 1 CUP

½ cup canola oil

¼ cup red wine vinegar

¼ cup water

2 tablespoons Italian seasoning

1 teaspoon granulated garlic

1 teaspoon lemon juice

1 teaspoon granulated onion

1 tablespoon dried vegetable flakes

Place all ingredients in a blender and pulse 2 to 3 times to combine.

PER 2 TABLESPOONS: Calories: 130 | Fat: 15g | Protein: 0g | Sodium: 320mg | Fiber: 0g | Carbohydrates: 1g

Mexican Ranch Dressing

A low-fat favorite with the added bonus of some zip.

INGREDIENTS | YIELDS 2 CUPS

1½ cups low-fat buttermilk salad dressing

Juice of 1 lime

1 tablespoon cilantro, chopped

1 teaspoon ground cumin

1 teaspoon chili powder

½ teaspoon ground coriander

¼ teaspoon dry mustard

Fresh cracked black pepper, to taste

1. Combine all ingredients in a bowl and mix to combine.

2. Allow to sit 10 minutes for flavor to develop before serving.

PER 2 TABLESPOONS: Calories: 50 | Fat: 4g | Protein: 0g | Sodium: 200mg | Fiber: 0g | Carbohydrates: 4g

Orange Juice Dressing

Orange juice makes a great base for dressings and marinades because it is fat free, flavorful, and a great complement to salads and meat.

INGREDIENTS | YIELDS 2¼ CUPS

1 cup fresh orange juice

¼ cup cold water

¼ cup canola oil

½ teaspoon ground ginger

2 tablespoons red wine vinegar

Zest of 1 orange

½ teaspoon red chili flakes

1. Place all ingredients except zest and chili flakes in blender. Blend for 1 minute to combine.

2. Add zest and chili flakes to blended mixture. Mix well.

3. Shake before using.

PER 2 TABLESPOONS: Calories: 35 | Fat: 3g | Protein: 0g | Sodium: 0mg | Fiber: 0g | Carbohydrates: 1g

Roasted Garlic Marinade

Rich with a touch of sweetness to add a depth of flavor without added fat.

INGREDIENTS | YIELDS 1½ CUPS; SERVING SIZE 1 TEASPOON PER 4 OUNCES OF MEAT

3 heads roasted elephant garlic

¼ cup canola oil

1 teaspoon cracked black pepper

¼ teaspoon salt

3 tablespoons balsamic vinegar

1. Peel roasted garlic out of skins and place pulp in bowl.

2. Add remaining ingredients and mix well to combine.

3. Store chilled and covered until ready to use.

PER TABLESPOON: Calories: 35 | Fat: 2.5g | Protein: 0g | Sodium: 25mg | Fiber: 0g | Carbohydrates: 3g

Taco Seasoning

Store brands are loaded with salt and sugar, but that is not the case with this tasty substitute. Combine with one pound of cooked lean beef for guilt-free tacos.

INGREDIENTS | YIELDS 1 CUP

4 tablespoons chili powder

1 teaspoon garlic powder

2 teaspoons onion powder

⅛ teaspoon cayenne

1 teaspoon cumin

1 teaspoon coriander

1 tablespoon Ancho chili powder

¼ teaspoon black pepper

½ teaspoon kosher salt

1 tablespoon Mrs. Dash's Bold and Spicy (or another low-sodium spice blend)

Mix all ingredients to combine and store in airtight container until ready to use.

PER RECIPE: Calories: 160 | Fat: 7g | Protein: 6g | Sodium: 1560mg | Fiber: 15g | Carbohydrates: 28g

Tuscan Herb Rub

More flavor, less salt, and the warm feelings of a Tuscan sunset.
Great on all types of meat and can also be used as a seasoning for roasted vegetables.

INGREDIENTS | YIELDS ½ CUP; SERVING SIZE 1 TEASPOON PER 4 OUNCES OF MEAT

2 tablespoons Italian seasoning

2 tablespoons fat-free grated Parmesan

2 tablespoons canola oil

1 tablespoon extra-virgin olive oil

¼ teaspoon cracked pepper

⅛ teaspoon red chili flakes

2 tablespoons balsamic vinegar

1 teaspoon summer savory, crushed

Mix all ingredients to combine and store in airtight container until ready to use.

PER TEASPOON: Calories: 20 | Fat: 2g | Protein: 0g | Sodium: 25mg | Fiber: 0g | Carbohydrates: 1g

Yogurt Marinade

Yogurt is flavorful and fat free, and it adds protein to this marinade.

INGREDIENTS | YIELDS 3 CUPS

2 cups fat-free plain yogurt

¼ yellow onion, thinly sliced

1 English cucumber, peeled, seeded, and thinly sliced

2 tablespoons fresh lime juice

3 sprigs fresh mint leaves, crushed

¼ cup skim milk

½ teaspoon red chili flakes

½ teaspoon black pepper

Mix all ingredients to combine and store chilled for one day before use.

PER RECIPE: Calories: 350 | Fat: 1.5g | Protein: 32g | Sodium: 410mg | Fiber: 3g | Carbohydrates: 53g

Red Wine Vinaigrette Dressing and Marinade

This salad dressing does double duty as both a dressing and marinade.
Just be sure to shake it before use so that the flavors are completely blended.

INGREDIENTS | YIELDS ½ CUP

¼ cup red wine vinegar

2 tablespoons orange juice

1 teaspoon sugar

½ teaspoon dry mustard

¼ teaspoon salt

1 teaspoon olive oil

1 scallion, chopped

1. Place all ingredients in a bowl and whisk until combined. Add salt and pepper to taste.

2. Store in airtight container in the refrigerator until ready to use.

PER RECIPE: Calories: 80 | Fat: 5g | Protein: 1g | Sodium: 580mg | Fiber: < 1g | Carbohydrates: 9g

Thai Peanut Sauce

Peanut sauce is normally very high in fat and sugar. This version has the same
great peanut taste without added oil or sugar. Use it to coat your cooked chicken
breast, then toss pasta with the remaining sauce and serve.

INGREDIENTS | YIELDS 1 CUP; SERVING SIZE 1 TABLESPOON PER 4 OUNCES OF MEAT OR PASTA

1 tablespoon orange juice concentrate

½ cup water

2 green onions, chopped

1 tablespoon ginger root, minced

1 tablespoon red pepper, minced

¼ cup natural or reduced-fat peanut butter

Juice of 1 lime

2 teaspoons low-sodium soy sauce

1 tablespoon rice wine

1. Combine orange juice concentrate and water in a small saucepan; bring to a simmer.

2. Add onions, ginger root, and red pepper. Cook until tender, approximately 7–8 minutes.

3. Remove from heat, whisk in peanut butter, lime juice, soy sauce, and rice wine. Use immediately or allow to cool and then refrigerate up to one week.

PER TABLESPOON: Calories: 30 | Fat: 1.5g | Protein: 1g | Sodium: 40mg | Fiber: 0g | Carbohydrates: 2g

Coconut Curry Sauce

This sauce is a great way to add great flavor to an otherwise boring chicken breast, featuring the Indian flavors of coconut and curry.

INGREDIENTS | YIELDS 2 CUPS; SERVING SIZE 2 TABLESPOONS

2 tablespoons yellow curry paste
2 tablespoons tomato paste
14 ounces unsweetened coconut milk
½ cup low sodium chicken stock
Juice of 1 lime
¼ cup cilantro leaves, chopped
2 tablespoons low-fat yogurt

1. In a sauté pan over medium heat, sauté curry paste and tomato paste for 1 minute.

2. Add coconut milk and chicken stock to pan; cook until it reduces by ⅓ in volume, about 10 minutes.

3. Add lime juice and cilantro; immediately remove from heat.

4. Whisk yogurt into sauce. Can be used immediately or refrigerated up to one week.

PER 2 TABLESPOONS: Calories: 50 | Fat: 5g | Protein: 1g | Sodium: 15mg | Fiber: 0g | Carbohydrates: 2g

Smoked BBQ Spice Rub

If you are planning to grill your meat, but you don't want the added sugar or calories of a BBQ sauce, try this smoky and savory spice rub for your chicken, pork, or beef.

INGREDIENTS | YIELDS ½ CUP

3 tablespoons smoked paprika
1 tablespoon black pepper
1 tablespoon celery seed
1 tablespoon sugar
1 tablespoon dry mustard
1 tablespoon onion powder
1½ tablespoons poultry seasoning
1 tablespoon dried thyme

1. Combine all ingredients and mix well. Rub generous amount of spice blend into meat.

2. Store any remaining rub in an airtight container.

PER SERVING: Calories: 260 | Fat: 7g | Protein: 9g | Sodium: 35mg | Fiber: 13g | Carbohydrates: 44g

Citrus Steak Rub

This spice rub has a hint of orange to complement the smoky flavors of chili and garlic. It is great for beef, pork, and chicken, on the grill or in the oven. This rub does not store well, so the recipe is just enough for a meal for two.

INGREDIENTS | YIELDS ¼ CUP

4 teaspoons garlic powder

2 teaspoons paprika

2 teaspoons dried orange peel

1 teaspoon chili powder

½ teaspoon black pepper

⅛ teaspoon kosher salt

Combine all ingredients and mix well. Rub generous amount of spice blend into meat.

PER SERVING: Calories: 70 | Fat: 1g | Protein: 3g | Sodium: 320mg | Fiber: 4g | Carbohydrates: 13g

Memphis Rub

This rub is a sweet and savory spice rub, reminiscent of the southern styles of BBQ that include sugar and molasses.

INGREDIENTS | YIELDS ½ CUP

¼ cup paprika

1 tablespoon packed dark brown sugar

1 tablespoon white sugar

1 teaspoon celery salt

1 teaspoon ground black pepper

1 teaspoon cayenne pepper, or to taste

1 teaspoon dry mustard

1 teaspoon garlic powder

1 teaspoon onion powder

1. Combine ingredients and mix well. Rub on pork or chicken, using a generous amount of spice blend.

2. Store in an airtight container.

PER SERVING: Calories: 230 | Fat: 4g | Protein: 6g | Sodium: 1030mg | Fiber: 10g | Carbohydrates: 46g

Chipotle Dry Rub

This spice blend is both smoky and spicy, but can be tailored to your individual tastes by adjusting the amount of chipotle peppers used.

INGREDIENTS | YIELDS ½ CUP

2 dried chipotle peppers

3 tablespoons black pepper

2 tablespoons dried oregano

1 tablespoon dried cilantro leaves

1 bay leaf

1 teaspoon cumin

1 teaspoon onion powder

1 teaspoon ground dry orange peel

1. Combine all ingredients in blender and process until ingredients are powdered. Rub on pork, beef, or chicken, using a generous amount of spice blend.

2. Store in an airtight container.

PER RECIPE: Calories: 160 | Fat: 3g | Protein: 5g | Sodium: 10mg | Fiber: 15g | Carbohydrates: 30g

Asian Dry Rub

If you enjoy pepper steak and other similar dishes in Asian restaurants, you will enjoy this rub, which combines tangy, sweet, and savory flavors.

INGREDIENTS | YIELDS ¼ CUP

1 tablespoon black peppercorns, crushed

¼ teaspoon salt

1 teaspoon brown sugar

½ teaspoon ground ginger

½ teaspoon ground cinnamon

1½ teaspoons anise seeds, crushed

¼ teaspoon ground cloves

1. Combine ingredients and mix well. Rub on pork, beef, or chicken, using a generous amount of spice blend.

2. Store in an airtight container.

PER RECIPE: Calories: 45 | Fat: 1g | Protein: 1g | Sodium: 590mg | Fiber: 2g | Carbohydrates: 10g

Mediterranean Spiced Chicken Marinade

If you are tired of baked chicken breast, this recipe is a flavorful solution to the boring chicken problem. Inspired by the flavors of North Africa, this recipe goes well with couscous or over rice pilaf.

INGREDIENTS | YIELDS 1 CUP; SERVING SIZE 1 TABLESPOON

1 tablespoon black pepper

1½ tablespoons paprika

1 teaspoon chili powder

1½ tablespoons garam masala

1 tablespoon ground cumin

1 tablespoon dried oregano

1 clove of garlic, chopped

1 teaspoon salt

2 tablespoons olive oil

4 tablespoons lemon juice

6 tablespoons fat-free yogurt

1. Combine all ingredients, stir until thoroughly blended.

2. Pour over chicken or pork and marinate in the refrigerator for at least 1 hour, but no longer than 8 hours.

PER TABLESPOON: Calories: 30 | Fat: 2g | Protein: <1g | Sodium: 150mg | Fiber: <1g | Carbohydrates: 2g

Jerk Chicken Marinade

This marinade is intense, dark in color, and has deep flavors and a little bit of spice to make it a savory delight.

INGREDIENTS | YIELDS 4 PORTIONS

1 tablespoon ground nutmeg

1 tablespoon ground allspice

1 tablespoon ground cinnamon

1 medium red onion, diced

3 green onions, chopped

¼ cup canola oil

1 cup orange juice

¼ cup low-sodium soy sauce

¼ cup fresh thyme

Juice of 1 lime

3 garlic cloves, smashed

1 jalapeño

2 inches ginger root, peeled and minced

Combine all ingredients in a food processor and process until smooth.

PER PORTION: Calories: 200 | Fat: 15g | Protein: 2g | Sodium: 540mg | Fiber: 4g | Carbohydrates: 18g

Mango Salsa

Cool and fruity, this salsa uses "slow" sugar to make it sweet without causing dumping syndrome. It also features fresh fruits and vegetables, which add fiber to your diet in a tasty way.

INGREDIENTS | YIELDS 4 PORTIONS

2 tablespoons honey

3 tablespoons lime juice

1 tablespoon ginger, minced

1 fresh mango, peeled and diced

½ cup cantaloupe, peeled, seeded, and diced

¼ cup red onion, diced

¼ cup red bell pepper, diced

1 English cucumber, diced

1 bunch cilantro

Combine all ingredients and mix well. Can be served immediately, but has better flavor if refrigerated overnight.

PER PORTION: Calories: 140 | Fat: 0g | Protein: 1g | Sodium: 15mg | Fiber: 2g | Carbohydrates: 35g

Mojo Marinade

This recipe uses garlic, citrus juices, and a variety of seasonings to take your chicken, beef, pork, or even seafood to another level.

INGREDIENTS | YIELDS 2½ CUPS

¼ cup garlic, chopped

½ cup yellow onion, chopped

2 cups fresh orange juice

½ cup lime juice

¼ cup canola oil

2 teaspoons salt

1 tablespoon black pepper

2 teaspoons ground cumin

2 teaspoons dried oregano

1 tablespoon fresh cilantro, chopped

1. Preheat large sauté pan over medium heat.

2. Combine all ingredients and pour into heated pan. Cook for 5 minutes.

3. Pour cooked mixture into a blender and pulse 3 to 4 times until chunky.

4. Chill for 1 hour before using. Store covered. Discard any excess marinade that comes into contact with raw meat.

PER 2 TABLESPOONS: Calories: 45 | Fat: 3g | Protein: 0g | Sodium: 230mg | Fiber: 0g | Carbohydrates: 4g

Peach Salsa

A departure from the standard tomato salsa, this salsa goes well with chicken and pork, or makes a great snack with tortilla chips.

INGREDIENTS | YIELDS 2 CUPS

½ tablespoon brown sugar

½ teaspoon allspice

¼ teaspoon cardamom ground

2 fresh ripe peaches, pitted and halved

¼ small red onion diced

Juice and zest from 1 orange

¼ red pepper, diced

¼ small jalapeño

Salt and pepper, to taste

⅛ cup chopped chervil

1. In a small bowl, mix brown sugar, allspice, and cardamom.

2. Dip the cut face of each peach in brown sugar mixture.

3. Place peaches face down on grill or heated surface until caramelized, about 4–5 minutes.

4. Dice the cooked peaches. Add to remaining ingredients and toss to combine.

5. Serve warm over pork chops or meat of your choice.

PER RECIPE: Calories: 230 | Fat: 1.5g | Protein: 5g | Sodium: 10mg | Fiber: 7g | Carbohydrates: 57g

Sweet Salsas

If you enjoy sweet salsas, consider making this one with fresh apricots, mangos, or fresh plums. For a crunchy treat, use diced jicama instead of peaches, as jicama is similar in texture to water chestnuts.

Chili Sauce

This chili sauce isn't overly spicy, but it does add a tremendous amount of flavor and a little bit of heat to pork.

INGREDIENTS | YIELDS ¾ CUP

½ cup fresh orange juice

¼ cup low-sodium Asian fish sauce

1 tablespoon low-sodium soy sauce

1 fresh Thai chili, seeded and minced

2 teaspoons Splenda

1 shallot, minced

1 tablespoon cilantro, chopped

1 green onion, chopped

½ teaspoon sesame seeds, toasted

Whisk together all ingredients. Allow to sit for 1 hour before using.

PER SERVING: Calories: 150 | Fat: 1.5g | Protein: 8g | Sodium: 6,100mg | Fiber: 2g | Carbohydrates: 30g

Red Pepper Sauce

Roasted red peppers have a more intense and smoky flavor than standard red peppers. Use this sauce on fish and chicken to heighten the flavor of your low-fat proteins.

INGREDIENTS | YIELDS 16 OUNCES; SERVING SIZE ¼ CUP

1 (12-ounce) can roasted red bell peppers

½ cup chicken stock

¼ teaspoon cumin

¼ teaspoon dry thyme

⅛ teaspoon cayenne

Juice from 1 lime

Salt and pepper, to taste

1. Place all ingredients, except the salt and pepper, in a small saucepan and bring to a simmer.

2. Once simmering, pour into a blender and blend until smooth. Return mixture to pan.

3. Season with salt and pepper to taste and garnish over fish or meat of your choice and serve.

PER ¼ CUP SERVING: Calories: 60 | Fat: 0g | Protein: 2g | Sodium: 450mg | Fiber: 0g | Carbohydrates: 9g

CHAPTER 16

Poultry

African Chicken and Rice

Low-fat chicken recipes have a tendency to be dry and bland. To replace the flavor lost from fat, this recipe uses chilies, tomatoes, and chicken stock to increase the flavor and keep the chicken moist.

INGREDIENTS | SERVES 6

1 tablespoon vegetable oil

¼ teaspoon dried thyme

1 clove garlic, crushed

2 pounds boneless skinless chicken breast

1 cup canned diced tomato

2 tablespoons tomato paste

1 medium onion, diced

1 quart low-sodium chicken stock

2 tablespoons ground dried shrimp

½ serrano chili, seeded and diced

1 cup white rice, cooked

1. Heat vegetable oil in a large pan over medium heat.

2. Mix thyme and garlic and rub mixture into the chicken.

3. Add diced tomato, tomato paste, and onion to heated oil and cook until clear and tender, about 3–4 minutes. Add the chicken and brown on all sides, 2–3 minutes per side.

4. Add stock, dried shrimp, and chili and cook at a strong simmer for 15 minutes.

5. Serve chicken on the rice and garnish with sauce.

PER SERVING: Calories: 410 | Fat: 8g | Protein: 51g | Sodium: 170mg | Fiber: 2g | Carbohydrates: 32g

Chicken Stock

Store-bought varieties of chicken stock are available in low-fat and low-sodium varieties. Start your recipes with a low-fat and low-sodium variety, then season your individual serving with salt if necessary. You'll eliminate unneeded fat and salt this way, and you will never even notice the change.

Buffalo Wings

Buffalo wings don't have to be greasy and deep fried to be tasty. This recipe is flavorful, the chicken is moist, and there is no added fat.

INGREDIENTS | SERVES 4

12 jumbo chicken wings, skin removed

1 tablespoon black peppercorns

1 medium onion

1 stalk of celery

1 head of garlic, halved

1 batch Hot and Spicy Marinade (page 193)

2 tablespoons Creole seasoning or spicy rub

Chicken Wings

Using this recipe as a guide, you can make low-fat chicken wings in a wide variety of flavors. Experiment with teriyaki, BBQ, ranch, citrus, and garlic marinades for interesting flavors without the fat.

1. Place chicken wings in a heavy deep pot and add peppercorns, onions, celery, and garlic; cover with cold water and bring to a simmer over medium heat and cook for 10–12 minutes.

2. Remove chicken from water and cool.

3. Coat in Hot and Spicy Marinade and let sit overnight.

4. Preheat oven to 350°F.

5. Spray sheet pan with nonstick spray and lay wings in a single layer on pan.

6. Sprinkle with Creole seasoning and roast in oven for 10–12 minutes until browned and cooked through. Serve with celery sticks and low-fat blue cheese dressing.

PER SERVING: Calories: 180 | Fat: 5g | Protein: 21g | Sodium: 1,180mg | Fiber: 2g | Carbohydrates: 12g

Tandoori Chicken

Love Indian food, but you aren't sure about the ingredients or if it is appropriate for your new diet? Try making this tandoori dish at home and you'll have the flavors of India without wondering if your diet has gone off track.

INGREDIENTS | SERVES 4

4 chicken thigh/leg quarters

4 tablespoons vegetable oil

2 teaspoons salt

1 teaspoon curry powder

1 teaspoon paprika

1 teaspoon turmeric

1 teaspoon ground coriander

1 teaspoon chili powder

1 teaspoon allspice

1 teaspoon ground ginger

1 teaspoon fresh chopped parsley

1 teaspoon garlic powder

2 tablespoons plain yogurt

1 fresh lime

1. Preheat oven to 375°F. Line a sheet pan with foil and place baking rack over foil.

2. Pull skin from chicken to bottom of leg (do not remove).

3. Combine all ingredients (except lime) and rub a thin coating onto chicken, then replace skin and place chicken on baking rack.

4. Cook 50–60 minutes until done, then squeeze fresh lime juice over chicken before serving.

PER SERVING: Calories: 290 | Fat: 24g | Protein: 16g | Sodium: 1,230mg | Fiber: 1g | Carbohydrates: 4g

Chicken Skin Is Bad?

Boiling the chicken before preparing the recipe helps remove the vast majority of fat from the skin of the chicken. If you are concerned about the fat that is left, feel free to remove the skin, but be aware that this chicken is very tender and may not retain its shape without the chicken skin in place.

Chicken Lettuce Wraps

The chicken lettuce wraps that you order in restaurants are usually loaded with fat and even higher in calories. This recipe removes almost all of the fat and replaces it with intensely flavorful ingredients that are healthy and combine for a restaurant-quality experience.

INGREDIENTS | SERVES 6

¼ cup low-sodium soy sauce

3 tablespoons garlic, minced

3 tablespoons ginger root, minced

¼ cup rice wine vinegar

1 teaspoon cilantro

2 tablespoons apricot all fruit preserves

2 teaspoons Asian chili paste

1 tablespoon canola oil

1 small carrot, diced

½ stalk celery, diced

¼ bell pepper, diced

5 snap peas, diced

¼ cup red onion, diced

½ cup fresh bean sprouts

2 chicken breasts, cut into small cubes

6 iceberg lettuce cups

2 tablespoons green onion, diced

2 tablespoons peanuts, toasted and crushed

5 wonton skins, baked crisp and crumbled

1. Combine soy, garlic, ginger, red wine vinegar, cilantro, apricot all fruit, and chili paste in a large pan and bring to a simmer to combine flavors.

2. In medium sauté pan heat oil over high heat. Add carrots, celery, bell pepper, snap peas, red onion, and bean sprouts; sauté for 45 seconds to 1 minute.

3. Add chicken and cook for 1–2 minutes, until chicken is no longer pink; add apricot sauce from large pan and simmer until chicken is cooked and tender (2–3 minutes).

4. Spoon into lettuce cups, garnish with green onion, peanuts, and crushed wontons.

PER SERVING: Calories: 140 | Fat: 5g | Protein: 12g | Sodium: 340mg | Fiber: 2g | Carbohydrates: 12g

Lettuce Wraps

Consider using lettuce wraps for other types of sandwiches, such as chicken salad. Lettuce is nearly calorie-free, but adds a crispness and crunch to your meal.

Jerk Chicken and Rice with Mango Salsa

This recipe uses the mango salsa recipe to balance out the intense flavors of jerked chicken with the citrus flavors of mango. This recipe is great for company, who will think you've become a gourmet chef. They will never know the dish is low in fat!

INGREDIENTS | SERVES 8

1 recipe of Jerk Chicken Marinade (page 201)

2 pounds boneless, skinless chicken breast, cubed

1 tablespoon oil

2 cups cooked rice

1 recipe of Mango Salsa (page 202)

1. Add chicken to Jerk Chicken Marinade in zip-top bag and place in refrigerator overnight.

2. Heat large pan and add 1 tablespoon oil. Add chicken and cook for 2 minutes per side until done.

3. Place on bed of cooked rice and top with Mango Salsa.

PER SERVING: Calories: 420 | Fat: 14g | Protein: 38g | Sodium: 360mg | Fiber: 3g | Carbohydrates: 37g

Rice Varieties

Rice is available in an amazing array of colors, flavors, and textures. Look at your local health food or Asian supermarket for rice in orange, red, black, and even purple colors.

Chicken Salad

Chicken salad in restaurants tends to be high in fat, loaded with mayonnaise and sour cream. This recipe removes the added fat but keeps the flavor that you love.

INGREDIENTS | SERVES 2

8 ounces cooked boneless skinless chicken breast, cut in small cubes

2 tablespoons fat-free mayonnaise

1 tablespoon low-fat sour cream

12 red seedless grapes, halved

3 tablespoons onion, minced

3 tablespoons celery, minced

1 teaspoon curry powder

1 teaspoon honey

Juice of 1 lime

Mix all ingredients together, chill, and season with salt and pepper to taste.

PER SERVING: Calories: 260 | Fat: 6g | Protein: 36g | Sodium: 220mg | Fiber: 1g | Carbohydrates: 15g

BBQ Pulled Chicken

Enjoy the flavor of southern BBQ without refined sugar and fat. If you are sensitive to sugar, the "slow" sugars in this recipe are usually better tolerated and shouldn't contribute to dumping syndrome.

INGREDIENTS | SERVES 6

1 tablespoon canola oil

1 large yellow onion, chopped

3 cloves garlic, minced

2½ cups low-sodium ketchup

¼ cup tomato paste

½ cup Diet Coke

⅓ cup apple cider vinegar

¼ cup molasses

¼ teaspoon black pepper

2 tablespoons dry mustard

½ teaspoon liquid smoke

1 (3-pound) roasted chicken, meat pulled off and shredded, skin removed

1. Heat oil in skillet over medium heat, add onions, and cook until soft (about 5 minutes), then add garlic and cook 1 minute.

2. Add ketchup, tomato paste, Coke, vinegar, molasses, pepper, mustard, and liquid smoke and bring to a boil, then reduce heat and allow to simmer for 15 minutes.

3. Add shredded chicken and cook for 10 more minutes, then place on your favorite toasted bun and enjoy.

PER SERVING: Calories: 410 | Fat: 9g | Protein: 48g | Sodium: 930mg | Fiber: 1g | Carbohydrates: 32g

BBQ Everything!

This sauce can be used on everything from roasted chicken to pulled pork. Try it on your favorite shredded beef, slather it on pork chops, or add some flavor to your baked chicken breast.

Nut-Crusted Chicken Breasts

It tastes like fried chicken, only it is low in fat and doesn't go anywhere near a fryer.

INGREDIENTS | SERVES 4

2 boneless, skinless chicken breasts, lightly pounded to even thickness

¼ cup flour

3 ounces liquid egg replacement

Salt and pepper, to taste

¼ teaspoon cinnamon

¼ teaspoon dry thyme

¼ teaspoon dry mustard

⅛ teaspoon cayenne

½ cup very finely chopped pistachios, walnuts, almonds, or pecans

2 tablespoons canola oil

4 tablespoons maple syrup

1 tablespoon Dijon mustard

Egg Replacements

If you are concerned about cholesterol and fat, replace the eggs you use for cooking and baking with egg replacements. They can be found in the frozen food department and in the egg area at your supermarket.

1. Preheat oven to 350°F.

2. Lightly dust chicken in flour and coat in beaten egg replacement.

3. In a medium bowl, combine salt and pepper, cinnamon, thyme, dry mustard, and cayenne with the chopped nuts.

4. Dredge (dip) chicken into nut mixture and press to completely cover the chicken.

5. Place oil in nonstick pan and heat over medium heat.

6. Place chicken in pan and cook until nuts brown (2–3 minutes), flip and cook for 2–3 minutes on second side, then place chicken in oven for 5–7 minutes.

7. In a small bowl, combine maple syrup and Dijon mustard. Pour over chicken for the last 2 minutes in the oven.

PER SERVING: Calories: 320 | Fat: 16g | Protein: 20g | Sodium: 170mg | Fiber: 2g | Carbohydrates: 25g

Chicken and Veggie Unfried Rice

Craving fried rice but you know that any food that starts with the word "fried" can't be a good fit for your diet? Try this low-fat recipe that has all of the best parts of fried rice without the calories or fat you find in restaurants.

INGREDIENTS | SERVES 4

Unflavored cooking spray

3 ounces liquid egg replacement

2 chicken breasts, cut into thin strips

1 garlic clove, minced

¼ teaspoon garlic chili paste

½ cup frozen mixed vegetables, thawed

½ yellow onion, finely chopped

¼ cup fresh bean sprouts

1 tablespoon low-sodium soy sauce

½ teaspoon sesame oil

2 cups cooked brown rice, cold

Add Some Veggies!

If you love your vegetables, or if you have trouble getting enough into your diet, consider adding a cup or two of steamed, chopped vegetables to this dish. Carrots, broccoli, edamame, and other vegetables work beautifully in this recipe.

1. Spray nonstick pan with spray; add liquid eggs and cook over low heat until a single sheet of cooked egg forms (like an omelet)—finish in oven if needed.

2. Pull eggs out and allow to cool, then fold over and cut into strips.

3. Heat pan and spray with cooking spray, add chicken, garlic, and chili paste and cook 2–3 minutes until almost done.

4. Add frozen vegetables, onion, and bean sprouts and cook another 2 minutes.

5. Add rice, soy sauce, and sesame oil, toss to heat, then add in the egg strips last, tossing to combine. Serve hot.

PER SERVING: Calories: 220 | Fat: 3g | Protein: 19g | Sodium: 170mg | Fiber: 3g | Carbohydrates: 27g

Rosemary Braised Chicken with Mushroom Sauce

The word "sauce" should set off warning bells for dieters everywhere. Sauces are usually fatty, loaded with salt, or have enough calories to make a meal by themselves. This sauce is one exception to the rule.

INGREDIENTS | SERVES 4

1 pound boneless skinless chicken thighs

2 tablespoons canola oil

2 slices turkey bacon or turkey prosciutto

1 small shallot, diced

¼ cup yellow onion, diced

1 clove garlic, crushed

3 sprigs fresh rosemary

3 ounces fresh cremini mushrooms, quartered

1 portobello mushroom cap, halved and sliced

1 teaspoon flour

1 cup low-sodium vegetable stock

½ cup red wine

Salt and pepper, to taste

1. Lightly coat chicken with oil, place in deep-sided skillet over medium heat, and brown on all sides (approximately 5 minutes per side).

2. Add bacon, shallots, onions, garlic, rosemary, and mushrooms, and sauté for 10 minutes.

3. Add flour, stock, and red wine; cover and reduce liquid by half until thick and chicken is cooked (approximately 10 minutes).

4. Serve chicken thighs sliced and covered with sauce. Season with salt and pepper to taste.

PER SERVING: Calories: 380 | Fat: 21g | Protein: 33g | Sodium: 260mg | Fiber: <1g | Carbohydrates: 9g

Portobello Mushrooms

Portobello mushrooms are an incredibly versatile vegetable. Marinated and grilled, they make a fantastic substitute for hamburgers, and cut into strips and sautéed they are a great side dish for your beef recipes.

Roast Turkey Breast

Roasted turkey breast is a naturally lean meat, but it also tends to be dry.
This recipe keeps your turkey moist and flavorful without adding butter.

INGREDIENTS | SERVES 12

1 onion

3 celery stalks

2 carrots

1 orange, sliced, skin on

2 large sprigs thyme

2 large sprigs rosemary

1 bone-in turkey breast from a 12–16 pound bird

1 tablespoon canola oil

Does Turkey Make You Sleepy?

Turkey does contain a chemical called tryptophan, which can help make people sleepy; however, most people are sleepy after a big turkey dinner because they ate too much! Don't eliminate turkey as a possibility for meals just because it has a bad reputation for causing a need for naps, just keep your portion size under control and there won't be a problem!

1. Cut onion, celery, and carrots in chunks.

2. Place chunks with orange slices, thyme, and rosemary in bottom of a roasting pan.

3. Coat turkey breast with oil and favorite rub. Place in roasting pan on top of vegetables—meat side down

4. Place in 425°F oven for 35 minutes.

5. Turn over turkey and reduce heat to 375°F. Cook for 1½ hours or until internal temp is 165°F. Check turkey every 15 minutes after first hour is past.

6. Remove turkey from oven and allow it to rest for 10 to 15 minutes on cutting board. Carve and serve. Great to use for sandwiches or in place of roast chicken.

PER SERVING: Calories: 180 | Fat: 2g | Protein: 35g | Sodium: 80mg | Fiber: 1g | Carbohydrates: 5g

Chicken Tacos

Skip the trip to a fast food restaurant and enjoy these tasty, diet-friendly tacos instead!

INGREDIENTS | YIELDS 6 TACOS

8 ounces ripe plum tomatoes, cored

2 teaspoons canola oil

8 ounces boneless chicken breast, cut into 1-inch chunks

Salt and pepper, to taste

½ teaspoon cumin

½ teaspoon chili powder

¾ cup yellow onion, chopped

1 clove garlic, minced

1 small chili pepper, seeded and diced

1 tablespoon lime juice

1 tablespoon chopped cilantro

6 corn tortillas, warmed

2 green onions

⅛ cup low-fat sour cream

¼ cup low-fat or fat-free Cheddar cheese

1. Heat large skillet on high heat until very hot. Place tomatoes in pan, turning regularly to char all sides, about 10 minutes.

2. Cut tomatoes in half and squeeze out seeds. Chop pulp and skin roughly, and set aside.

3. Reduce heat and add oil to pan. Add chicken and season with salt and pepper, cumin, and chili powder.

4. Cook chicken until brown on all sides, about 5 minutes.

5. Add onions, pepper, garlic, lime juice, and cilantro. Cook for 2 minutes.

6. Add prepared tomatoes and simmer until hot and chicken is cooked.

7. Place on warm tortillas and garnish with green onions, sour cream, and cheese.

PER TACO: Calories: 170 | Fat: 5g | Protein: 16g | Sodium: 100mg | Fiber: 3g | Carbohydrates: 17g

Curried Chicken Meatballs with Rice

If you like curry, these chicken meatballs are a real treat. Packed with the protein you need, these meatballs also have the flavor you crave.

INGREDIENTS | SERVES 4

1 pound lean ground chicken
½ cup yellow onion, minced
¼ cup cilantro, chopped
3 tablespoons low-fat plain yogurt
3 tablespoons flour
¼ teaspoon cumin
¼ teaspoon turmeric
¼ teaspoon ground coriander
¼ teaspoon garam masala
1 small serrano chili, seeded and diced
2 cloves garlic, minced
¼ cup egg substitute
½ recipe Coconut Curry Sauce (page 198)

1. Preheat oven to 350°F.

2. Combine all ingredients and mix well.

3. Scoop into 2-ounce portions and form into balls.

4. Place meatballs on sprayed sheet pan and bake for 7 minutes.

5. Place curry sauce in saucepan over medium heat and bring to a simmer.

6. Coat cooked meatballs with curry sauce and serve over rice.

PER SERVING: Calories: 210 | Fat: 10g | Protein: 22g | Sodium: 105mg | Fiber: <1g | Carbohydrates: 9g

Meatballs!

If you love meatballs but you aren't a huge fan of curry, try swapping the coriander, garam masala, and turmeric for onion powder, garlic powder, and a low-salt seasoning blend. Swap the fresh cilantro for fresh parsley and you have a brand new meatball recipe.

Chicken Pasta Salad

Great use of leftover chicken with great flavor and very little fat.

1. Cook pasta according to directions on box and rinse to cool.

2. Mix cooled pasta with remaining ingredients to combine and serve chilled.

PER SERVING: Calories: 340 | Fat: 15g | Protein: 21g | Sodium: 310mg | Fiber: 3g | Carbohydrates: 29g

Oven-Roasted Mojo Chicken

This recipe uses the Mojo Marinade (page 202) to create a flavorful chicken dish. High in protein and low in fat, this recipe is quick and easy, and reheats well.

Short on Time?

You can chop the chicken and have this recipe in the oven in less than 5 minutes when you make the marinade the night before.

1. Pour marinade over chicken and let sit overnight.

2. Preheat oven to 375°F.

3. Place onions, tomatoes, and okra on sheet pan. Place chicken skin side up on top of vegetables

4. Pour remaining marinade over chicken and place in oven.

5. Cook for 75 minutes until crispy and done. Serve over rice with pan juices.

PER SERVING: Calories: 340 | Fat: 9g | Protein: 54g | Sodium: 360mg | Fiber: 1g | Carbohydrates: 8g

Roasted Chicken

A tasty low-fat version of roasted chicken that has many uses.

INGREDIENTS | YIELDS 1 CHICKEN; SERVES 8

1 medium yellow onion, peeled and chopped

2 stalks celery, chopped roughly

1 medium carrot, peeled and chopped

1 head garlic, cut in half

1 sprig fresh thyme

1 sprig fresh rosemary

1 teaspoon kosher salt

½ teaspoon black pepper

1 teaspoon garlic powder

1 teaspoon onion powder

2 tablespoons canola oil

1 (3½-pound) chicken, skin removed, rinsed and dried

1. Preheat oven to 350°F.

2. Place chopped vegetables and herbs in bottom of roasting pan.

3. In a small bowl, combine oil and spices. Rub mixture on all surfaces of chicken.

4. Place chicken on top of vegetables breast side down and cover. Cook for 35 minutes.

5. Flip over chicken in pan. Cook uncovered for another 45 minutes.

6. When internal temperature is 155°F, or chicken is fully cooked at the joints, remove from oven and allow to rest. Carve and serve.

PER SERVING: Calories: 240 | Fat: 8g | Protein: 35g | Sodium: 440mg | Fiber: <1g | Carbohydrates: 5g

Roasted Chicken Galore

You can use your leftover roasted chicken in a multitude of ways. Consider using it for chicken salad, chicken soup, or chicken sandwiches. You can make chicken tacos, chicken potpies, or even top a heart-healthy pizza with it!

CHAPTER 17

Pork and Beef

Beef Kabobs

Love your steak but worry about portion control? These kabobs are four ounces of beef along with some fresh fruit and vegetables to offer a complete meal with minimal fuss.

INGREDIENTS | SERVES 4

4 bamboo or metal skewers

8 medium mushroom caps, marinated for 24 hours with meat in 1 recipe Roasted Garlic Marinade (page 195)

1 red bell pepper, cut in strips

1 pound cubed stew meat (marinated for 24 hours in Roasted Garlic Marinade)

1 small red onion, quartered, with the root end still attached

1 cup fresh pineapple cubes

1 ounce low-sodium soy sauce

1 tablespoon honey

1. Soak wooden skewers in water for 30 minutes.

2. Place mushroom cap on skewer, then peppers, meat (about 4 ounces per skewer), onion, pineapple, and finish with another mushroom cap.

3. In a small bowl, combine soy sauce and honey. Brush mixture onto kabobs.

4. Grill kabobs over open grill until done, approximately 3 minutes per side or bake on rack in a 375°F oven for 6 minutes. Serve with rice.

PER SERVING: Calories: 230 | Fat: 8g | Protein: 26g | Sodium: 380mg | Fiber: 2g | Carbohydrates: 15g

Lamb or Beef Stew with Apricots and Saffron

Apricots give this recipe its sweetness, saffron gives it a beautiful color. This is not your average stew, but it is a diet-friendly one. You can also substitute beef for the lamb if you desire.

INGREDIENTS | SERVES 6

1½ pounds cubed lamb stew meat

2 tablespoons canola oil

1 medium onion, sliced

3 cloves of garlic, smashed

1 cinnamon stick

½ teaspoon saffron

1 tablespoon flour

1¼ cups low-sodium beef stock

1½ cups dried apricots, soaked in warm water until plump and chopped into pieces

Salt and pepper, to taste

1½ teaspoons Tabasco

1. Sear lamb in sauté pan with oil until browned.

2. Add onions and garlic and sauté until browned, about 3–4 minutes.

3. Add cinnamon and saffron and cook for 2 minutes.

4. Add in flour, stir to combine. Add in stock and apricots and simmer for 1 hour until meat is tender.

5. Remove cinnamon stick. Season with salt and pepper and Tabasco and serve over couscous.

PER SERVING: Calories: 300 | Fat: 11g | Protein: 25g | Sodium: 100mg | Fiber: 3g | Carbohydrates: 25g

Turkey Bacon–Wrapped Beef Tenderloin

You don't have to give up the great flavor of beef tenderloin when you are trying to lose weight, you just have to be careful about your portion size and how the meat is prepared.

INGREDIENTS | SERVES 2

Cooking spray
4 strips turkey bacon
2 (4-ounce) beef tenderloins
1 tablespoon crushed peppercorns
1 cup sliced mushrooms
1 clove garlic, smashed
1 teaspoon dry thyme
1 tablespoon flour
3 ounces red wine
3 ounces low-sodium beef stock

Beef Tenderloin

Beef tenderloin is one of the leanest cuts of beef available, making it a great addition to your diet, as long as you stay away from traditional preparations like covering it with butter or hollandaise.

1. Spray medium-sized sauce pan with cooking spray, then heat over medium heat until hot.

2. Wrap bacon around tenderloin and secure with a toothpick.

3. Roll tenderloins (bacon side out) in peppercorns and sear for 3 minutes per side for medium doneness.

4. Remove meat from pan and cook mushrooms and garlic in the pan for 3 minutes.

5. Add flour and red wine and thyme, and simmer for 3–4 minutes until reduced by ¾.

6. Add stock and simmer 3–4 minutes until thickened.

7. Add tenderloins back to sauce for 1 minute and serve hot.

PER SERVING: Calories: 400 | Fat: 25g | Protein: 29g | Sodium: 360mg | Fiber: 2g | Carbohydrates: 8g

Pork Tenderloin with Cherry Sauce

Pork tenderloin is a great way to feed your family, because it is perfectly sized to make a meal for four. Tenderloin is also a very lean cut of pork, making it a great choice for your diet.

INGREDIENTS | SERVES 4

1 pound pork tenderloin (not pork loin)

¼ teaspoon salt

¼ teaspoon freshly ground black pepper

2 sliced shallots

1 teaspoon olive oil

½ cup dried cherries

1 cup low-sodium chicken stock

3 tablespoons balsamic vinegar

1 teaspoon tarragon

¼ cup pomegranate juice

Tasty Tenderloin

Consider baking your tenderloin, then slathering it with barbecue sauce for a tasty treat. You can coat the entire tenderloin, or you can slice it then coat each slice with barbecue sauce for more intense flavor.

1. Preheat oven to 350°F.

2. Lightly season pork with salt and pepper and sear in a large sauté pan. Place in oven to roast for 10 to 15 minutes (until internal temperature reaches 155°F). Remove pork from oven and allow meat to rest.

3. Meanwhile, place shallots, oil, and cherries in a sauce pan and cook for 2 minutes.

4. Add remaining ingredients and bring to a boil.

5. Simmer 10–12 minutes until cherries break down and liquid reduces.

6. Slice pork and garnish with sauce.

PER SERVING: Calories: 280 | Fat: 6g | Protein: 26g | Sodium: 230mg | Fiber: < 1g | Carbohydrates: 32g

Braised Pork Burritos

Don't go out for burritos that are covered in cheese, slathered with sour cream, and cooked with enough oil to ruin your diet for days. Instead, try this lean but tasty recipe with restaurant flavor and diet-conscious calories.

INGREDIENTS | YIELDS 12 BURRITOS

2 pounds pork loin, trimmed of visible fat

Cooking spray

1 medium yellow onion, diced

2 cloves garlic, minced

1 medium apple, peeled and diced

1 cup water

1 tablespoon apple cider vinegar

3 pounds diced fresh tomatoes

1 small cinnamon stick

⅓ teaspoon ground cloves

⅓ cup golden raisins

8–12 tortilla shells

⅓ cup toasted almonds

Salt and pepper, to taste

Pulled Pork

This recipe can make a barbecue version of pulled pork if you are looking for something sweet instead of savory. Follow the recipe, then add the barbecue sauce of your choice to the shredded pork and serve on buns.

1. Preheat oven to 350°F.

2. Coat oven-safe sauté pan (with a lid) with cooking spray, then warm over medium-high heat. Once pan is hot, cook pork on each side for 2 minutes.

3. Add onions to pan and cook until onions are clear, approximately 4 minutes.

4. Add garlic, apples, water, and vinegar, stirring continuously for two minutes, scraping the bottom of the pan.

5. Add tomatoes, cinnamon, cloves, and salt and pepper to taste.

6. Cover pan and move it to the oven. Simmer in oven until pork is tender, approximately 1 hour. Add raisins in the last few minutes of cooking.

7. Remove pork and shred with forks. Add back to pan and mix with other ingredients.

8. Fill tortilla shells with pork mixture, garnish with almonds, and serve.

PER SERVING: Calories: 280 | Fat: 12g | Protein: 24g | Sodium: 105mg | Fiber: 4g | Carbohydrates: 20g

Mini Meat Loaf

This recipe is full of lean protein, but even better, you can make it in advance, freeze it, and pull it out when you just don't feel like cooking.

INGREDIENTS | SERVES 4

4 ounces lean ground beef

4 ounces lean ground pork

4 ounces lean ground chicken

1 small egg, beaten

⅛ cup instant oatmeal

⅛ cup parsley

1½ tablespoons skim milk

½ medium onion, chopped fine

Salt and fresh ground black pepper, to taste

⅛ cup ketchup

¾ teaspoon Worcestershire sauce

Freezing for Later

If you have made these meat loaves ahead and frozen them, add half an hour to the cooking time to make sure it is thoroughly cooked. Test the meat loaf with a knife to make sure it is hot all the way through, slice, and serve.

1. Preheat oven to 375°F.

2. Mix all ingredients except ketchup and Worcestershire sauce in mixing bowl to combine.

3. Spray mini loaf pans or muffin tins with nonstick cooking spray, portion meat into 4 equal parts, and fill pans.

4. In a small bowl, mix ketchup and Worcestershire sauce to form a glaze. Brush onto the top of each loaf.

5. Bake 25–30 minutes until done.

6. Pour off extra fat and serve.

PER SERVING: Calories: 190 | Fat: 11g | Protein: 17g | Sodium: 170mg | Fiber: < 1g | Carbohydrates: 6g

Asian Flank Steak with Edamame and Soba

If you enjoy the flavors of Asia, this dish includes sesame, teriyaki, and chili paste.
Low in fat, but high in protein, fiber, vitamins, and minerals, this recipe is a diet dream.

INGREDIENTS | SERVES 4

¼ pound soba noodles

1 teaspoon canola oil

4 ounces trimmed beef flank steak, sliced thinly across grain

1½ tablespoons lime juice

1½ tablespoons low-sodium teriyaki sauce

1½ tablespoons garlic and chili paste

½ teaspoon cornstarch

½ teaspoon sesame oil

½ red pepper, julienned

2 green onions, diagonally cut

8 snow peas, cut into strips

¼ cup shredded carrot

1 cup frozen edamame, thawed

1 tablespoon fresh minced ginger root

¼ cup cilantro

1. Cook soba noodles according to package directions.

2. While noodles are cooking, heat sauté pan with oil. Add steak to pan and cook until just done (approximately 2 minutes). Remove steak from pan and set aside, keeping warm.

3. Whisk lime juice, teriyaki, chili paste, ginger root, cornstarch, and sesame oil together to form a sauce.

4. Add red pepper, onions, snow peas, and carrot to pan and add prepared sauce. Cook 2 minutes.

5. Add beef and juices from plate back into pan. Add edamame, toss to heat through.

6. Add soba noodles and toss. Garnish with fresh cilantro, and serve.

PER SERVING: Calories: 230 | Fat: 4g | Protein: 17g | Sodium: 370mg | Fiber: 3g | Carbohydrates: 31g

Soba Noodles

Soba noodles are noodles made from buckwheat. They are more flavorful than standard pasta and also tend to be higher in fiber and protein. If you don't have them at your local store, they can be found easily online, or you can substitute standard pasta.

Country Spare Ribs with White Beans

Country spare ribs are naturally low in fat and high in protein but can be very dry if overcooked. Cooking the ribs slowly means they are tender and moist but still tasty and diet appropriate.

INGREDIENTS | SERVES 8

2 pounds lean country pork ribs
¼ cup canola oil
½ cup red peppers, diced
1 cup diced onion
½ cup celery, diced
2 tablespoons flour
1 tablespoon diced garlic
1 cup canned diced plum tomatoes
½ cup dried navy beans
4 cups vegetable stock
1 tablespoon Dijon mustard
1 tablespoon garlic powder
2 tablespoons Worcestershire sauce
1 tablespoons dried oregano
2 sprigs fresh thyme
1 bay leaf
1 teaspoon salt
1 teaspoon fresh ground black pepper
Steamed brown rice

1. Preheat oven to 350°F.

2. Place ribs on sheet pan in oven and cook 10 minutes per side to render fat and brown.

3. Heat Dutch oven. Add oil, peppers, onions, and celery. Cook about 6–7 minutes or until onions are clear.

4. Add flour and stir. Add garlic and beans, place ribs on top. Pour stock, tomatoes, mustard, garlic powder, Worcestershire, oregano, thyme, bay leaf, salt, and pepper over ribs.

5. Place Dutch oven in oven and simmer ribs and beans for 1½–2 hours, stirring every 15 minutes.

6. Serve over brown rice.

PER SERVING (WITHOUT RICE): Calories: 390 | Fat: 18g | Protein: 30g | Sodium: 1,120mg | Fiber: 8g | Carbohydrates: 30g

Pork Chops with Peach Salsa

Pork and peaches are a perfect compliment. If you are tired of baked pork and looking for something just as healthy with a lot of flavor, this is the recipe you've been looking for.

INGREDIENTS | SERVES 2

2 boneless center-cut pork chops, approximately 4 ounces each

Salt and pepper, to taste

2 tablespoons Chinese Five-Spice Rub (page 191)

½ cup orange juice

1 recipe of Peach Salsa (page 203)

1. Preheat oven to 350°F. Spray an oven-safe pan with cooking spray, heat pan over medium heat.

2. Rub pork chops with Chinese Five-Spice Rub and place in pan.

3. Cook for 3 minutes until browned; flip and repeat.

4. Add orange juice. Move pan to oven for 4–6 minutes.

5. Garnish with generous portion of Peach Salsa, salt and pepper to taste.

PER SERVING: Calories: 340 | Fat: 9g | Protein: 28g | Sodium: 55mg | Fiber: 4g | Carbohydrates: 41g

Grilled Pork Skewers with Chili Dipping Sauce

Naturally lean pork tenderloin adds protein to your diet, and the spicy dipping sauce makes it intensely flavorful.

INGREDIENTS | SERVES 6

¼ cup low-sodium soy sauce

¼ cup low-sodium teriyaki sauce

3 tablespoons cilantro, chopped

2 tablespoons garlic, chopped

2 tablespoons Splenda

1 teaspoon black pepper

2 tablespoons lime juice

1½ pounds pork tenderloin, cut into 16 long strips

16 bamboo skewers, soaked in water

1 recipe Chili Sauce (page 204)

2 cups cooked rice

1. Whisk all liquids together, then add garlic, cilantro, Splenda, and pepper; stir to combine. Pour over pork. Marinate for 2 hours.

2. Put one piece of meat on each skewer, laying it flat.

3. Heat griddle pan on high heat and cook pork for 3 minutes per side.

4. Serve with Chili Sauce and rice.

PER SERVING (WITHOUT RICE): Calories: 180 | Fat: 4g | Protein: 26g | Sodium: 1,600mg | Fiber: < 1g | Carbohydrates: 9g

Pork Shoulder Roast

This portion is large enough for a small dinner party. The roast will shrink by about half after cooking, leaving two to three pounds of flavorful but inexpensive pork roast.

INGREDIENTS | SERVES 12

2 tablespoons fresh sage, chopped

2 tablespoons fresh rosemary, picked and chopped

10 cloves garlic, minced

1 tablespoon fennel seeds, toasted

1½ tablespoons kosher salt

1 tablespoon black pepper

1 tablespoon orange juice

2 cups apple cider

1 pork shoulder roast, 4 to 5 pounds, tied by butcher

3 Granny Smith apples, cut in half and cored

Extra Servings

If you don't have a large family or feel like having a dinner party, this pork shoulder freezes well, and also makes tasty sandwiches, pulled pork, and quesadillas. It can also make a lovely addition to a hearty bean soup.

1. Preheat oven to 275°F.

2. Combine sage, rosemary, garlic, fennel, salt, pepper, orange juice, and apple cider in food processor and blend into a paste.

3. Rub paste all over pork roast.

4. Place apples in roasting pan, rest roast on top of them.

5. Cover and cook for 6 hours on middle rack of oven.

6. When internal temperature reaches 175°F and the meat shreds with a fork, remove from oven and allow to rest for 15 minutes.

7. Shred meat with fork and serve.

PER SERVING: Calories: 310 | Fat: 12g | Protein: 38g | Sodium: 1030mg | Fiber: 1g | Carbohydrates: 11g

Tequila Lime London Broil

*London broil doesn't usually conjure up thoughts of lime and tequila,
but this recipe combines the two with lean meat to make a terrific dinner.*

**INGREDIENTS | YIELDS 12 (4-OUNCE)
PORTIONS**

1 jalapeño, seeded

1 clove garlic, smashed

1 cup tequila

1 cup low-sodium soy sauce

2 tablespoons sesame oil

¼ cup Worcestershire sauce

¼ teaspoon kosher salt

¼ teaspoon black pepper

¼ cup lime juice

1 medium onion, peeled and chopped

3½ pounds trimmed London Broil

1. Combine all ingredients except beef in blender and puree.

2. Pour resulting sauce over beef in nonreactive container and marinate for 3 hours.

3. Heat grill pan on high heat and cook meat 4 to 5 minutes per side. Turn meat 4 times while cooking. When done, remove from heat and allow to rest 10 minutes.

4. Make sure to cut thin slices across the grain of the meat.

PER SERVING: Calories: 290 | Fat: 12g | Protein: 29g |
Sodium: 890mg | Fiber: 0g | Carbohydrates: 4g

Pizzaiola Steaks

*This is a low-fat, high-flavor steak entrée that manages
to sneak in some heart-healthy vegetables.*

INGREDIENTS | SERVES 4

4 (4-ounce) sliced rump or chuck steaks

Salt and pepper, to taste

3 tablespoons flour

3 tablespoons canola oil

3 cloves garlic, smashed

1 (14-ounce) can plum tomatoes with
juice, chopped

2 tablespoons fresh basil, chopped

2 cups packed baby spinach

1. Dredge steaks in flour to coat and tap to remove excess. Lightly season with salt and pepper.

2. Heat nonstick pan over medium heat and add oil and garlic. Cook for 1 minute.

3. Raise heat to high and add steaks to pan. Brown steaks quickly on both sides.

4. Add in tomatoes, basil, and spinach. Reduce heat to low and simmer 12 to 15 minutes covered.

PER SERVING: Calories: 320 | Fat: 19g | Protein: 25g |
Sodium: 105mg | Fiber: 2g | Carbohydrates: 11g

Spinach

Spinach is high in iron, vitamin C, and
antioxidants.

Roast Pork Loin with Rosemary and Garlic

This pork loin is tasty enough to be served at a dinner party,
but healthy enough to make a regular appearance on your dinner table.

INGREDIENTS | SERVES 8

3 tablespoons chopped fresh rosemary, or 1 tablespoon dried

4 cloves garlic, minced

1 teaspoon kosher salt, divided

½ teaspoon freshly ground pepper, plus more to taste

1 (2-pound) boneless center-cut pork loin roast, visible fat trimmed

4 teaspoons extra-virgin olive oil, divided

1. Preheat oven to 400°F.

2. In a small bowl, combine rosemary, garlic, salt, and pepper. Mix thoroughly.

3. Coat baking dish with cooking spray. Place pork in the dish and rub the rosemary mixture on the meat.

4. Place the dish in the oven and roast the pork for 30 minutes.

5. Remove the pan from the oven. Carefully turn the pork over.

6. Roast the pork for another 30 minutes or until a meat thermometer inserted into the pork reads 145°F. Remove from heat and allow the pork to rest for at least 10 minutes.

7. Slice the pork and serve.

PER SERVING: Calories: 290 | Fat: 18g | Protein: 30g | Sodium: 360mg | Fiber: 0g | Carbohydrates: 1g

CHAPTER 18

Fish and Seafood

Grilled Crab Legs

Do you love crab legs but you know that the way you usually eat them, drenched in butter, isn't such a good idea? Grilling crab legs intensifies the flavor so you don't need butter to make them tasty.

INGREDIENTS | YIELDS 4 (1-CLUSTER) PORTIONS

4 large claw clusters of crab legs (Snow crab or King crab)

Lemon juice, to taste

Butter Substitute

If crab legs just don't seem like crab legs without the butter flavor, try using butter spray. You can find it where you find butter in your local grocery store, but it is nearly free of calories and very low in fat.

1. Soak crab legs in water for half an hour.

2. Place crab legs on a hot charcoal or gas grill. Cook for 3 minutes per side until shells turn a dusty orange color and water stops bubbling from the shells.

3. Squeeze fresh lemon juice over meat and enjoy.

PER SERVING: Calories: 25 | Fat: 0g | Protein: 6g | Sodium: 105mg | Fiber: 0g | Carbohydrates: 0g

Shrimp and Vegetable Kabob

Shrimp is wonderful for someone who is trying to watch what they eat. Naturally low in fat, shrimp is a high-protein treat that doesn't need butter or oil to taste great.

INGREDIENTS | YIELDS 4 KABOBS

8 peeled and deveined (16/20) jumbo shrimp, tails removed, soaked in Citrus Marinade (page 192) for 20 minutes

4 skewers (bamboo or metal)

1 red bell pepper

1 cup pineapple, cubed

1 small red onion, quartered with root end attached

1. Place shrimp and veggies on skewers alternating meat and fruit.

2. Place on barbecue grill, grill pan, or in oven (preheated to 350°F) for 3 minutes per side.

3. Brush with marinade twice while cooking, once per side until done.

PER SERVING: Calories: 120 | Fat: 7g | Protein: 4g | Sodium: 25mg | Fiber: 1g | Carbohydrates: 11g

Salmon with Red Pepper Sauce

Salmon is naturally high in antioxidants and omega-3 fatty acids, which can actually help lower your bad cholesterol and raise your good cholesterol.

INGREDIENTS | SERVES 2

1 tablespoon olive oil

Salt and pepper, to taste

2 (4 ounce) skinned salmon fillets

1 recipe Red Pepper Sauce (page 204)

1. Heat nonstick pan over medium heat, add oil, and heat 1 minute.

2. Season fish with salt and pepper and place round side down for 4 minutes.

3. Flip fish and cook for 4 more minutes for medium fish doneness.

4. Remove fish from pan and allow it to rest for 2 minutes before garnishing with the Red Pepper Sauce and serving.

PER SERVING: Calories: 440 | Fat: 12g | Protein: 30g | Sodium: 1,860mg | Fiber: 0g | Carbohydrates: 34g

Seared Tuna with White Bean Salad

Love tuna but tired of tuna salad? Try this seared tuna for a new way to eat this diet-friendly fish.

INGREDIENTS | SERVES 2

2 (4-ounce) fresh ahi tuna steaks

1 tablespoon prepared basil pesto

1 teaspoon canola oil

Salt and pepper, to taste

½ red bell pepper, seeded and julienned

½ green bell pepper, seeded and julienned

¼ red onion, thinly julienned

¼ cup shredded carrot

¼ cup Kalamata olives

½ cup plum tomatoes, seeded and diced

½ cup prepared low-fat balsamic vinaigrette

½ cup fresh basil leaves, torn

1. Rub tuna with pesto and let sit for 1 hour.

2. Heat nonstick pan over medium-high heat and add oil.

3. Season tuna with salt and pepper, then place in hot oil and cook 1½ to 2 minutes per side for medium rare. Remove from pan and place on plate.

4. Combine all remaining ingredients (except basil) and toss in hot pan for 30–45 seconds to heat through, then add basil and pour over tuna.

PER SERVING: Calories: 390 | Fat: 15g | Protein: 36g | Sodium: 1,200mg | Fiber: 3g | Carbohydrates: 25g

Seared Scallops with Apricot Orzo Salad

Scallops make a great addition to a healthy diet plan. Low in fat, high in protein, scallops are a flavorful way to increase the protein in your plan.

INGREDIENTS | SERVES 3

1½ cups cooked orzo

3 tablespoons dried cherries

¼ cup chopped dried apricots

2 tablespoons toasted pine nuts

Salt and pepper, to taste

1 teaspoon canola oil

6 large U/10 dry-packed scallops

1. Cook orzo according to package directions.

2. Place cherries and apricots in a strainer and pour boiling water from orzo over them to soften and drain.

3. Once drained, combine with pine nuts and salt and pepper to taste.

4. Heat skillet over high heat and add canola oil, heating until smoking.

5. Season scallops with salt and pepper, place in hot oil, cook 2 minutes and turn, cooking an additional 2 minutes over medium-high heat.

6. Place on plate and serve with orzo salad.

PER SERVING: Calories: 380 | Fat: 16g | Protein: 13g | Sodium: 50g | Fiber: 3g | Carbohydrates: 48g

Halibut En Papillote

Baking fish in parchment paper allows it to cook quickly, sealing in all of the flavor, and leaving the fish tender.

INGREDIENTS | SERVES 2

1 medium shallot, sliced into rings

1 teaspoon garlic, minced

1 tablespoon canola oil

2 teaspoons capers

¼ cup fresh tomato, diced

2 sprigs fresh tarragon

½ cup julienned carrots

½ cup julienned red bell peppers

½ cup julienned celery

½ cup julienned leeks

½ cup julienned yellow squash

¼ cup low-sodium vegetable stock

2 (4-ounce) portions halibut

1. Preheat oven to 450°F.

2. For each portion, cut a large circle out of parchment paper, fold in half, place fish in the seam and put mixed vegetables and herbs. Drizzle oil over the top of each portion.

3. Pour 2 tablespoons of stock on each and seal the edges of the paper by folding it over and crimping.

4. Place on a sheet pan in oven for 12–14 minutes, then serve on a bed of rice or couscous.

PER SERVING: Calories: 250 | Fat: 10g | Protein: 26g | Sodium: 320mg | Fiber: 3g | Carbohydrates: 15g

En Papillote

En papillote, or "in paper," is a classic French method of food preparation. Best used with fish and other seafood, cooking in paper is not only flavorful, but can make a dramatic presentation at dinner and also allows for quick and easy cleanup.

Roasted Black Cod with Mushrooms and Potatoes

Black cod is more flavorful than other types of cod, even though it is low in fat.
If you enjoy fish, try this sustainable North Atlantic variety.

INGREDIENTS | SERVES 4

Cooking spray

1¾ pounds Yukon Gold potatoes, cut into ½-inch-thick rounds

Salt and pepper, to taste

1 tablespoon canola oil

2 cloves garlic, smashed

½ pound fresh mushrooms, mixture of shiitake, cremini, portobello, etc.

4 (6-ounce) black cod fillets

Juice from 1 lemon

Chopped parsley, for garnish

About Black Cod

Black cod is a North Atlantic fish that is stronger in flavor than other types of cod, but it is hardier than many types of fish, enough to stand up to roasting. Try black cod seared or grilled for a change of pace.

1. Preheat oven to 475°F.

2. Line large roasting pan with waxed paper, put potatoes in a single layer in the pan and drizzle with oil, then cook for 18–20 minutes until golden.

3. Coat sauté pan with cooking spray. Add mushrooms and garlic and sauté until lightly cooked; pour over potatoes.

4. Season fish with salt and pepper and place on top of mushrooms and potatoes skin side up and drizzle with a touch of oil.

5. Bake for 10 minutes, remove from oven, squeeze lemon juice on top, add parsley, and serve.

PER SERVING: Calories: 540 | Fat: 30g | Protein: 29g | Sodium: 110mg | Fiber: 3g | Carbohydrates: 38g

Tuna Pasta Salad

This recipe is high in protein and low in fat, with a potent lemon flavor.

INGREDIENTS | SERVES 8

8 ounces bow tie pasta

2 tablespoons canola oil

1 can spring water–packed tuna

2 cups canned cannellini beans, drained and rinsed

½ small red onion, cut into thin rings

1 celery stalk, sliced into thin half moons

1 tablespoon lemon juice

1 tablespoon chopped parsley

Salt and pepper, to taste

1. Cook pasta according to directions on package. Rinse under cold water and drain well.

2. Combine all ingredients in a bowl and lightly toss to combine. Allow to sit 1 hour before serving.

PER SERVING: Calories: 210 | Fat: 5g | Protein: 13g | Sodium: 200mg | Fiber: 3g | Carbohydrates: 28g

Shrimp Salad

Shrimp salad doesn't have to be loaded with mayonnaise or dressing to taste great. Try this version compatible with a low-fat diet and you'll find you don't miss the fat.

INGREDIENTS | SERVES 2

8 ounces peeled and deveined 26/30 shrimp, tails removed and cooked

1 tablespoon Dijon mustard

1 teaspoon honey

¼ cup sweet corn kernels

1 tablespoon lemon juice

¼ cup red bell pepper diced

2 tablespoons low-fat sour cream

¼ cup diced tomatoes

¼ cup diced red onions

¼ teaspoons horseradish

½ tablespoon chopped chervil

Combine all ingredients. Season to taste with salt and pepper.

PER SERVING: Calories: 200 | Fat: 5g | Protein: 25g | Sodium: 370mg | Fiber: 2g | Carbohydrates: 15g

Shrimp and Cholesterol

If you are watching your cholesterol, you may want to limit the amount of shrimp you eat each week. Shrimp is high in cholesterol, so try to limit your intake to 2 or 3 servings per week if your cholesterol is elevated.

Seared Salmon with Peppercorn Sauce

This isn't your everyday salmon: With a splash of brandy and a hint of spice, this salmon is a great meal for a date who will never suspect it is low in fat.

INGREDIENTS | SERVES 2

2 (5-ounce) salmon fillets

1 teaspoon each green, black, and pink peppercorns, crushed

1 tablespoon canola oil

1 shallot, minced

2 tablespoons brandy

½ teaspoon fresh dill, chopped

½ teaspoon fresh thyme, picked and chopped

½ cup prepared low-sodium veal demi-glace

1. Preheat oven to 350°F.

2. Place salmon fillet face down in crushed peppercorns to coat.

3. Heat nonstick pan over medium high heat and add oil.

4. Place fish peppercorn side down in pan and cook for 3 minutes.

5. Flip fillet and cook 3 more minutes then place in oven for 4 minutes.

6. Add shallots and brandy to sauté pan (be careful, it may flame).

7. Cook until reduced by half (approximately 5 minutes) and add remaining ingredients. Season to taste.

8. Pour over fish and serve.

PER SERVING: Calories: 280 | Fat: 12g | Protein: 29g | Sodium: 170mg | Fiber: 0g | Carbohydrates: 4g

Stewed Mussels and Clams with Tomatoes and Olives

This dish is both easy and quick, but has the flavor of a dish that took hours to prepare.

INGREDIENTS | SERVES 4

¾ pound fresh mussels, shell on

¾ pound fresh clams, shell on

2 tablespoons canola oil

3 cloves garlic, smashed

¼ cup white wine

1 tablespoon lemon juice

½ cup black olives, pitted

1 cup fresh plum tomatoes, diced

1 cup low-sodium vegetable or seafood stock

Zest of 1 lemon

⅛ teaspoon red chili flakes

5 tablespoons fresh parsley, chopped

1. Soak clams and mussels in cold running water to clean. Discard any open or broken shells.

2. Heat oil in sauté pan over medium heat, add garlic and chili flakes. Cook 1 minute and increase heat to high.

3. Add remaining ingredients except parsley and cover. Steam for 5 to 8 minutes until shellfish are open.

4. Pour into bowl, add parsley, and serve with crusty bread.

PER SERVING: Calories: 250 | Fat: 12g | Protein: 23g | Sodium: 530mg | Fiber: 1g | Carbohydrates: 10mg

Grilled Swordfish with Lemon, Capers, and Olives

Grilled swordfish is often called the steak of the sea, so if you are trying to limit the amount of red meat that you eat, try cooking this fish instead.

INGREDIENTS | SERVES 4

1 tablespoon canola oil

2 tablespoons lemon juice

½ red Thai chili, seeded and chopped

4 (6-ounce) swordfish fillets

Zest of 1 lemon

1 clove garlic, chopped

2½ tablespoons capers, drained and rinsed

10 Kalamata olives, roughly chopped

2 tablespoons red onion, finely chopped

2 tablespoons low-fat Parmesan cheese, shredded

1. Preheat grill pan over high heat.

2. In a bowl combine oil, lemon juice, and Thai chili and pour over swordfish.

3. In another bowl, combine zest, garlic, capers, olives, red onion, and Parmesan cheese, and mix well.

4. Place swordfish in hot pan and cook for 2 to 3 minutes per side.

5. Place on fish plate and spoon prepared relish over fish. Garnish with parsley if desired.

PER SERVING: Calories: 270 | Fat: 12g | Protein: 35g | Sodium: 450mg | Fiber: < 1g | Carbohydrates: 3g

Guilt-Free Comfort Food

Unfried Fried Chicken

Crispy fried chicken with only one tablespoon of added fat tastes great without loading you down with fat and calories.

INGREDIENTS | SERVES 8

1 tablespoon butter

1 cup flour

1 tablespoon granulated garlic

1 tablespoon onion powder

1 package buttermilk ranch dressing powder

½ teaspoon ground black pepper

1 teaspoon dried parsley flakes

1 teaspoon season salt

1 whole chicken (approximately 3 pounds), visible fat and skin removed, cut into 8 pieces

1. Preheat oven to 375°F.

2. Place heavy skillet in oven with butter in it.

3. Combine flour, garlic, onion powder, dressing powder, black pepper, parsley flakes, and salt in a bowl and mix.

4. Rinse chicken in water and dredge to coat in seasoning mix.

5. Place chicken "skin" side down in hot pan, bake for 30 minutes.

6. Turn the chicken and bake another 20 minutes until done and serve.

PER SERVING: Calories: 290 | Fat: 9g | Protein: 37g | Sodium: 280mg | Fiber: <1g | Carbohydrates: 13g

Tuna Noodle Casserole

Craving comfort food but avoiding unwanted fat and calories? Try this version of an old favorite.

INGREDIENTS | SERVES 6

6 ounces dried wide whole wheat egg noodles

2 teaspoons canola oil

½ cup softened, chopped sun-dried tomatoes, not oil packed

1 small onion, diced small

1 red bell pepper, diced small

1 clove minced garlic

1 stalk celery, diced

2 tablespoons all-purpose flour

2 cups skim milk

½ cup fat-free mayonnaise

1 can spring water–packed tuna, drained (or canned chicken)

½ cup grated low-fat Swiss cheese

2 tablespoons chopped fresh basil

1 tablespoon lemon juice

Salt and pepper, to taste

⅓ cup toasted almonds

1. Preheat oven to 425°F. Spray a quart casserole dish with nonstick cooking spray.

2. Cook pasta about 6 minutes, drain, rinse in cold water, and set aside.

3. Heat pan and add oil and garlic. Cook vegetables and tomatoes for 3 minutes.

4. Add flour. Cook for 1 minute.

5. Add milk. Bring to a boil and simmer for 4 minutes.

6. Stir in mayo, tuna, cheese, and basil.

7. Season with lemon juice, salt, and pepper.

8. Sprinkle with almonds and bake for 20 minutes. Let stand 5 minutes before serving.

PER SERVING: Calories: 310 | Fat: 9g | Protein: 23g | Sodium: 340mg | Fiber: 5g | Carbohydrates: 37g

Beefy Onion Belgian Stew

This beef stew is both hearty and healthy.

INGREDIENTS | SERVES 8

2 tablespoons canola oil

2 pounds lean stew meat, cubed

3 cloves garlic, smashed

Salt and freshly ground black pepper

1 cup low-sodium beef stock

1 small yellow onion, diced

2 cups light beer

1 tablespoon brown sugar

2 parsley sprigs

1 bay leaf

1 sprig fresh thyme

1 tablespoon red wine vinegar

1 tablespoon cornstarch

Skip the Can!

While canned beef stew is easy, it isn't nearly as tasty as this homemade version. Instead of buying stew at the grocery store, make this one ahead, and freeze individual portions ahead.

1. Preheat oven to 325°F.

2. In a heavy pan, heat oil and brown beef a few pieces at a time until nicely browned, approximately 3 minutes; remove beef.

3. Reduce heat and add onions. Cook until caramelized, about 10 minutes.

4. Add cooked beef and garlic and remaining ingredients; stir to deglaze pan.

5. Bring to a simmer. Cover and place in oven.

6. Braise until fork tender (about 60 to 75 minutes); skim off any fat.

7. Season and serve over whole wheat pasta or rice.

PER SERVING: Calories: 330 | Fat: 17g | Protein: 36g | Sodium: 90mg | Fiber: 0g | Carbohydrates: 4g

Pizza for One

Pizza doesn't have to be eliminated from your diet when you are trying to lose weight. This pizza can be part of your diet without slowing down your weight loss.

INGREDIENTS | SERVES 1

1 (6-inch) flour tortilla shell, or 6-inch round lavash cracker bread

Canola oil

4 tablespoons Tomato Sauce (page 254)

¼ cup low-fat shredded Mozzarella cheese

4 roasted garlic cloves, smashed

8 slices turkey pepperoni

4 basil leaves, fresh torn

Vegetables on Pizza

Do not overload pizza with lots of watery vegetables or the crust will not crisp. For a vegetable pizza, cook all vegetables first and drain, then place on the pizza before baking.

1. Preheat oven to 350°F.

2. Brush tortilla lightly with oil and bake for 3 minutes until crisp. (If using lavash, skip this step.)

3. Raise heat in oven to 375°F.

4. Brush on sauce, add garlic and pepperoni, top with cheese, then bake on a sheet pan or pizza stone until cheese melts and crust is crisp.

5. Garnish with torn basil and serve hot.

PER SERVING: Calories: 450 | Fat: 20g | Protein: 33g | Sodium: 1570mg | Fiber: 2g | Carbohydrates: 33g

Cabbage Rolls with Tomato Sauce

Cabbage rolls are hearty and filling, but low enough in calories to be eaten on a regular basis. Make these ahead and freeze them or feed a hungry group of people with this large recipe.

INGREDIENTS | YIELDS 1 DOZEN LARGE ROLLS

2 heads green cabbage

¼ cup canola oil

1 yellow onion, chopped

2 garlic cloves, chopped

1 ounce red wine vinegar

2 tablespoons tomato paste

2 tablespoons chopped parsley

½ cup tomato sauce

½ pound lean ground beef

½ pound lean ground pork

1 pound lean ground chicken

¼ cup egg substitute

1½ cups cooked rice

1 batch of Cabbage Roll Sauce (page 247)

1. Preheat oven to 350°F.

2. Break cabbage into large leaves and blanch in boiling water for 4 minutes.

3. In sauté pan cook onions and garlic in oil for 2 minutes, add vinegar, tomato paste, parsley, and tomato sauce, then mix to incorporate and remove from heat.

4. In a large bowl, mix meat, eggs, and rice with onion mixture.

5. Lay small leaves on bottom of casserole and spoon Cabbage Roll Sauce over to lightly coat, then take larger leaves with core removed and scoop in filling (approximately ½ cup each).

6. Roll like a burrito and tuck ends in, place seam side down and fill baking dish.

7. Cover with remaining 1 cup of sauce and bake for 45–60 minutes until meat is cooked.

PER ROLL: Calories: 360 | Fat: 16g | Protein: 18g | Sodium: 170mg | Fiber: 6g | Carbohydrates: 26g

Cabbage Roll Sauce

This tomato sauce perfectly complements cabbage rolls with a hint of garlic and caraway.

INGREDIENTS | YIELDS 1½ QUARTS; SERVES 12

2 tablespoons canola oil

2 garlic cloves, smashed

1½ quarts crushed tomatoes

2 tablespoons white vinegar

1 tablespoon stevia or Splenda

Salt and pepper, to taste

1 tablespoon caraway seeds, toasted and crushed

1. Combine all ingredients and simmer for 30 minutes.

2. Blend or puree until smooth and adjust seasoning.

> **PER RECIPE:** Calories: 50 | Fat: 2.5g | Protein: 1g | Sodium: 70mg | Fiber: 1g | Carbohydrates: 6g

Caraway Seeds

Caraway seeds are the seeds found in rye bread. They add a savory and earthy tone to food and go well with tomatoes, cabbage, and other vegetables. Try them sprinkled on your steamed vegetables to heighten the flavor without increasing the calories.

Potato Pancakes

Potato pancakes don't have to be smothered in oil to be crispy. In this recipe the combination of a small amount of butter and a nonstick pan are enough to produce a tasty pancake without frying.

INGREDIENTS | YIELDS 4 SMALL CAKES

1 large potato, peeled and shredded

¼ yellow onion, grated

1 ounce egg substitute

Pinch nutmeg

2 tablespoons flour

1 tablespoon fat-free Parmesan cheese

1 tablespoon dried chives

1 tablespoon butter, melted

Fresh ground black pepper

1. In a bowl, combine all ingredients to form a batter.

2. Spray a nonstick skillet with cooking spray and heat over medium heat.

3. Ladle ¼ cup of batter onto pan and cook until pancake is golden brown, approximately 4 minutes, then flip and continue to cook about 4 more minutes.

4. Serve with applesauce and low-fat sour cream.

> **PER PANCAKE:** Calories: 90 | Fat: 3.5g | Protein: 3g | Sodium: 40mg | Fiber: <1 g | Carbohydrates: 12g

Mashed Potatoes

Mashed potatoes can be creamy without butter, sour cream, or cream. This recipe uses low-fat ingredients to produce the creamy texture you crave.

INGREDIENTS | SERVES 6

1 pound peeled and cubed potatoes or 1 pound Yukon Gold potatoes with skins on

¼ cup plain silken tofu

½ cup fat-free or low-fat sour cream

2 tablespoons roasted garlic

½ cup skim milk

Salt and pepper, to taste

1 tablespoon dry chives

1. Boil potatoes until fork-tender, drain, then place in a mixer (or a large bowl and use a hand mixer) with the tofu, sour cream, and garlic. Whip until blended but do not over mix.

2. Add milk to thin slightly (may not need all of the milk) and add chives, stirring to combine.

3. Season and serve.

PER SERVING: Calories: 110 | Fat: 3g | Protein: 3g | Sodium: 25mg | Fiber: 1g | Carbohydrates: 18g

Stuffed Peppers

This recipe can easily be made vegetarian by replacing the ground turkey with cooked and seasoned rice.

INGREDIENTS | SERVES 6

6 large green or red bell peppers, tops removed and seeded

4 cups low-sodium vegetable stock

1 (28-ounce) can Italian tomatoes

2 medium zucchini, grated

½ cup low-fat Parmesan cheese

2 ounces canola oil

3 cloves garlic, minced

1 teaspoon salt

1 teaspoon black pepper

½ cup basil leaves

1 cup cooked orzo pasta

½ cup yellow onion, diced

1 pound ground turkey or chicken

1. Preheat oven to 400°F.

2. Place peppers in a 3-quart baking dish and pour vegetable stock into pan.

3. Crush or chop tomatoes and combine with the remaining ingredients and stuff peppers.

4. Cover with foil and bake for 45 minutes; uncover and bake for another 10–12 minutes.

5. Sprinkle with additional cheese to brown if desired.

PER SERVING: Calories: 390 | Fat: 17g | Protein: 23g | Sodium: 1,460mg | Fiber: 5g | Carbohydrates: 39g

Baked Beans

These beans are high in protein and fiber without any meat. If you are looking for a hearty and meatless dish, you've found it.

INGREDIENTS | SERVES 8

¾ cup dry pinto beans

¾ cup dry red kidney beans

¾ cup dry navy beans

5 cups low-sodium vegetable stock

1 medium onion peeled and halved

⅓ cup molasses

1 tablespoon Dijon mustard

1 teaspoon salt

½ cup chopped canned tomatoes

1 tablespoon apple cider vinegar

Bacon with Your Baked Beans?

If baked beans don't seem like baked beans without bacon on top, try covering the dish with turkey bacon. You get the flavor of bacon without the fat and calories. Liquid smoke can also add a more intense flavor without adding calories.

1. Soak beans overnight after picking and sorting.

2. Preheat oven to 250°F.

3. Drain beans and place in a large pot with vegetable stock, then bring to a boil over high heat and simmer for 30 minutes.

4. Drain and reserve stock.

5. Place beans in a 2½ quart baking dish with onion.

6. Mix remaining ingredients. Pour over beans, covering them completely, then cover dish and bake for 4 hours, checking every ½ hour and adding more reserved stock if needed.

PER SERVING: Calories: 250 | Fat: 1g | Protein: 13g | Sodium: 720mg | Fiber: 12g | Carbohydrates: 49g

Berry Cheese Blintzes

Blintzes don't need to be made with crepes to taste great. Using wonton wrappers keeps the fat content down while frozen berries keep them flavorful.

INGREDIENTS | SERVES 4 (2 PER PERSON)

1½ cups low-fat or fat-free ricotta cheese

½ cup low-fat or fat-free cream cheese

¼ cup egg substitute

3 tablespoons stevia or Splenda

1 orange zest, finely grated

1 package large round wonton wrappers (8 pieces)

2 tablespoons butter, melted

1 teaspoon vanilla extract

1 quart frozen berries (raspberries or strawberries)

¼ cup orange juice

¼ cup Splenda

1 teaspoon cornstarch

1. Preheat oven to 375°F.

2. Combine ricotta, cream cheese, vanilla, egg substitute, 3 tablespoons of Splenda, and zest in a bowl and mix to make filling.

3. Brush wonton skins with butter on both sides, divide the filling into 8 equal parts, and place on the lower ⅓ of the wonton skins.

4. Roll blintzes into neat packages (like a burrito) with ends tucked and seam side down onto nonstick sheet pan.

5. Bake until golden and crisp.

6. Take berries, Splenda, orange juice, and cornstarch and combine in a pan.

7. Bring to a boil and simmer until fruit is soft, then blend until smooth and serve over the blintzes.

PER SERVING: Calories: 380 | Fat: 19g | Protein: 18g | Sodium: 320mg | Fiber: 4g | Carbohydrates: 36g

Roasted Chicken and Vegetable Quesadillas

By using reduced-fat dairy products, this quesadilla is a healthy version with all of the flavor of the original.

INGREDIENTS | YIELDS 1 QUESADILLA

Nonstick cooking spray

2 (6-inch) flour tortillas

¼ cup low-fat pepper jack or Cheddar cheese

3 ounces roast chicken, diced

½ cup roast veggies, diced

1 ounce lettuce, shredded

2 tablespoons low-fat sour cream

¼ cup salsa or pico de gallo

1. Spray nonstick pan with cooking spray over medium heat; place 1 tortilla in pan and cover with ½ of the cheese.

2. Add chicken and veggies, and cover with remaining cheese.

3. Top with the second tortilla and cook until cheese melts and bottom tortilla crisps, then flip over and cook another 2–3 minutes.

4. Cut into wedges and garnish with lettuce, sour cream, and salsa.

PER SERVING: Calories: 520 | Fat: 14g | Protein: 48g | Sodium: 1,330mg | Fiber: 6g | Carbohydrates: 47g

Green Bean Casserole

This family favorite doesn't need fried onions to taste great. Bread crumbs and fresh onions give this casserole great flavor without frying.

INGREDIENTS | SERVES 8

½ yellow onion, sliced thin

2 tablespoons butter

1 cup bread crumbs

½ cup low-fat Parmesan cheese

1 cup low-fat or fat-free cream of mushroom soup

½ cup skim milk

1 teaspoon soy sauce

Fresh ground black pepper

4 cups cut green beans, frozen and thawed

1 tablespoon dry thyme

1. Preheat oven to 350°F.

2. Sauté onions in butter and add bread crumbs and Parmesan.

3. Mix all remaining ingredients together and pour into a casserole dish.

4. Cover with bread crumbs and onion mixture and bake for 20–25 minutes.

PER SERVING: Calories: 150 | Fat: 6g | Protein: 6g | Sodium: 390mg | Fiber: 3g | Carbohydrates: 20g

Ground Pork Wonton Ravioli

Low-fat ravioli have the same great taste when wonton wrappers are used instead of pasta and are stuffed with a tasty pork and shrimp blend.

INGREDIENTS | YIELDS 18 RAVIOLIS

8 ounces ground pork

4 ounces shrimp

1 green onion, finely chopped

2 garlic cloves, minced

1-inch fresh ginger root, peeled and minced

1 egg white

1 teaspoon cornstarch

1 teaspoon garlic chili paste

Juice of ¼ of a lemon

1 tablespoon low-sodium soy sauce

Pinch of salt and fresh ground black pepper

1 tablespoon ground shiitake mushrooms dried

2 drops toasted sesame oil

3 large Savoy cabbage leaves, shredded fine

36 round wonton wrappers

1. Place all ingredients except the cabbage and wrappers into a food processor and grind to form a paste.

2. Fold in shredded cabbage.

3. Place a wonton wrapper on cutting board or counter. Put 1 tablespoon of prepared filling in the center of wonton.

4. Brush cold water on edges of the wonton and cover with a second wonton. Carefully remove all air and seal edges.

5. Poach in water or stock until they float.

PER RAVIOLI: Calories: 70 | Fat: 3g | Protein: 5g | Sodium: 110mg | Fiber: 0g | Carbohydrates: 6g

Tasty Raviolis

You can serve these raviolis as an appetizer with a side of tomato sauce, make them into a full-fledged meal, or poach them in chicken stock instead of water to create a tasty soup.

Pasta with Spring Vegetables

Light flavors and crisp vegetables are the star of this low-fat, high-fiber entrée.

INGREDIENTS | SERVES 4

1 pound cooked pasta, such as penne or rotini

2 tablespoons canola oil

1 small carrot, peeled and cut into thin rounds

2 green onions, diced

2 medium tomatoes, diced

½ cup frozen peas

½ cup frozen cut green beans

1 small yellow bell pepper, diced

1 clove garlic, chopped

1 tablespoon butter

2 tablespoons low-fat Parmesan cheese

6 leaves fresh basil, torn

1. Cook pasta according to directions on box. Do not drain.

2. Heat large sauté pan and add oil.

3. Add carrots, onions, tomatoes, peas, green beans, yellow pepper, and garlic to the pan and sauté vegetables until tender, about 3 to 4 minutes.

4. Add pasta directly from boiling water to the pan. Add butter.

5. Toss to combine and sprinkle with Parmesan and basil.

PER SERVING: Calories: 620 | Fat: 19g | Protein: 19g | Sodium: 85mg | Fiber: 7g | Carbohydrates: 95g

Pasta with Alfredo Sauce

This sauce is a low-fat version of a high-fat classic pasta dish.

INGREDIENTS | SERVES 2

Nonfat cooking spray

2 cloves garlic, minced

2 tablespoons fat-free cream cheese

1⅓ cups skim milk

2 tablespoons all-purpose flour

2 tablespoons butter sprinkles (or butter substitute)

1 cup fat-free or low-fat Parmesan cheese

Black pepper, to taste

2 cups cooked pasta of choice

1. Spray nonstick skillet with cooking spray. Add garlic over low heat and cook until tender.

2. Add cream cheese, milk, and flour, whisking over medium heat; bring to a boil.

3. Reduce heat to a simmer and cook until sauce has thickened.

4. Add butter sprinkles, Parmesan cheese, and black pepper, whisk until combined. Immediately add to pasta and toss to coat.

PER SERVING: Calories: 440 | Fat: 1.5g | Protein: 27g | Sodium: 990mg | Fiber: 3g | Carbohydrates: 60g

Low-Fat, High-Flavor Quiche

A lower-fat version of a Sunday brunch favorite.

INGREDIENTS | SERVES 6

1 (9-inch) reduced-fat prepared pie crust
½ cup steamed vegetables
½ cup low-fat Cheddar cheese
¾ cup liquid egg replacement
½ cup fat-free milk
2 tablespoons fat-free sour cream
Pinch each of salt and pepper

1. Preheat oven to 350°F.

2. Place empty pie crust on center rack and bake for 5 to 6 minutes. Remove from oven.

3. Place vegetables and cheese in partially baked crust and spread out evenly.

4. Whisk egg replacement, milk, sour cream, salt, and pepper together.

5. Pour into shell and bake for 35 to 45 minutes until done.

PER SERVING: Calories: 170 | Fat: 9g | Protein: 8g | Sodium: 270mg | Fiber: < 1g | Carbohydrates: 15g

Tomato Sauce

This tomato sauce is a great way to top your pasta, without the sugar and other additives you will find in store-bought varieties.

INGREDIENTS | SERVES 8

1 medium onion, chopped
2 large cloves of garlic, peeled and chopped
1¼ cups water
1 (32-ounce) can Italian crushed tomatoes
1 teaspoon dried basil
1 teaspoon dried oregano
Pinch dried chili flakes
½ teaspoon salt

1. Place onion and garlic in sauce pan with ¼ cup of water. Sauté for 5 minutes, or until softened.

2. Add tomatoes, remaining water, basil, oregano, chili flakes, and salt to pan; cover and simmer for 30 minutes.

3. Blend for 30 seconds in a blender for a smooth sauce, or leave chunky.

PER SERVING: Calories: 45 | Fat: 0g | Protein: 2g | Sodium: 420mg | Fiber: 2g | Carbohydrates: 7g

Loaded Smashed Potato

Just because you have given up food that is loaded in fat doesn't mean you have to give up loaded baked potatoes. This recipe exchanges high-fat and high-calorie ingredients for low-fat substitutes without sacrificing flavor.

INGREDIENTS | SERVES 2

1 large Idaho baking potato

Cooking spray

Salt and pepper, to taste

2 tablespoons low-fat sour cream

1 tablespoon butter flakes

2 tablespoons low-fat Cheddar cheese

2 strips turkey bacon, cooked until crisp, crumbled

1 scallion, chopped

Butter Replacement

If you love butter but you know it isn't the best thing for your diet, consider the wide range of butter substitutes that are available. There are now butter sprays, flakes, and powders that have most of the flavor of butter, but none of the fat and few of the calories.

1. Preheat oven to 350°F.

2. Spray potato with cooking spray then sprinkle with salt and pepper. Place in oven and bake for 45 minutes or until fork-tender.

3. Once potato is cooked, cut in half lengthwise and scoop soft potato into a bowl, leaving the skin as a shell.

4. Add remaining ingredients in bowl, stir to combine.

5. Place half of the mixture in each potato skin shell, return to oven and bake for 5 additional minutes. Serve hot.

PER SERVING: Calories: 210 | Fat: 4.5g | Protein: 8g | Sodium: 250mg | Fiber: 4g | Carbohydrates: 36g

Baked Mac and Cheese

This favorite comfort food is no longer a diet disaster. You can indulge your love for creamy pasta without sacrificing your weight loss goals.

INGREDIENTS | SERVES 4

2 cups low-fat or fat-free ricotta cheese

1½ cups skim milk, divided use

1 tablespoon all-purpose flour

2 cups elbow macaroni, cooked

1½ cups low-fat or fat-free shredded mozzarella or Cheddar cheese

1 cup dry bread crumbs, toasted

Salt and pepper, to taste

1. Preheat oven to 350°F.

2. In a medium bowl, combine ricotta and ½ cup milk and blend until smooth.

3. In a separate bowl, combine flour and ¼ cup milk, blend until smooth.

4. Heat remaining milk in sauce pan until steaming, add ricotta and flour combinations, whisk until smooth and thickened.

5. Add pasta to milk and cheese mixture and toss.

6. Pour into baking dish, top with remaining cheese and bake for 25 minutes.

7. Sprinkle with bread crumbs, bake for additional 5 minutes or until crumbs are browned.

8. Add salt and pepper to taste, serve while hot.

PER SERVING: Calories: 580 | Fat: 11g | Protein: 35g | Sodium: 590mg | Fiber: 3g | Carbohydrates: 78g

Eggplant Lasagna

Craving lasagna? Try this low-fat recipe that is hearty and filling without the fat and calories you don't want. Using eggplant instead of pasta noodles keeps the calorie content down, but increases the fiber and adds flavor.

INGREDIENTS | SERVES 6

1 medium eggplant, cut into ¼ inch slices

2 tablespoons lemon juice

Cooking spray

2 cups tomato sauce

1 can whole tomatoes, drained and chopped

2 cloves garlic, minced

¼ teaspoon red chili flakes

1 tablespoon basil

1 tablespoon oregano

⅓ cup bread crumbs

¼ cup fat-free Parmesan cheese, grated

1 cup fat-free ricotta cheese

1 cup fat-free mozzarella cheese, shredded

Fat-Free Cheese

The flavor and texture of fat-free cheese has improved dramatically in recent years. It doesn't always melt as well as low-fat or regular cheese, but you can always substitute low-fat cheese for the fat-free cheese in this recipe if you are looking for a more gooey, melted consistency.

1. Preheat oven to 350°F.

2. Brush eggplant slices with lemon juice, place on baking sheet (after coating sheet with cooking spray). Cook until tender, approximately 10 minutes, turning after 5 minutes.

3. Combine tomato sauce, chopped tomatoes, garlic, chili flakes, oregano, and basil in a bowl. Set aside.

4. Combine Parmesan and bread crumbs in a bowl. Set aside.

5. Combine ricotta and mozzarella cheese in a bowl. Set aside.

6. Coat 9-inch square pan with cooking spray. Begin with a layer of the sauce mixture, then the eggplant slices, then ricotta and mozzarella cheese mixture. Repeat until all ingredients are used.

7. Spread bread crumb mixture over the top; bake for 45 minutes.

PER SERVING: Calories: 170 | Fat: 0.5g | Protein: 14g | Sodium: 410mg | Fiber: 5g | Carbohydrates: 24g

CHAPTER 20

Side Dishes

Green Lentil and Olive Salad

Tired of green salads as your side dish? Try this high-protein lentil salad for a savory change of pace.

INGREDIENTS | SERVES 6

Juice of 1 lemon

1 teaspoon Dijon mustard

1 tablespoon olive oil

1 cup green lentils, soaked and cooked until tender

2 tomatoes, diced

1 small red onion, diced

1 small serrano chili, seeded and diced

Salt and pepper, to taste

1 bunch fresh parsley, chopped

4 mint leaves, chopped

2 romaine lettuce crowns

1. In a small bowl, combine lemon juice, mustard, and olive oil to make dressing. Set aside.

2. Combine lentils, tomatoes, onion, chili, salt and pepper, parsley, and mint. Serve on the romaine lettuce and top with prepared dressing.

PER SERVING: Calories: 150 | Fat: 3g | Protein: 9g | Sodium: 45mg | Fiber: 8g | Carbohydrates: 24g

Sun-Dried Tomato Pesto

Standard pesto is one third oil and one third pine nuts, making it fatty and high in calories. This version omits the oil and reduces the amount of nuts, making it diet-friendly.

INGREDIENTS | YIELDS 2½ CUPS; SERVING SIZE ¼ CUP

2½ cups sun-dried tomatoes (not packed in oil)

3 cups boiling water

2 tablespoons pine nuts, toasted

2 cloves garlic, smashed

⅔ cup fresh basil

2 tablespoons low-fat or fat-free Parmesan cheese

¼ cup Italian parsley leaves

3 tablespoons white wine

1. Rehydrate tomatoes for 1 hour in boiling water. Drain the tomatoes but reserve the water.

2. Grind tomatoes, pine nuts, garlic, basil, Parmesan, and parsley in a food processor. Add wine with ½ of the remaining tomato water to thin.

PER ¼ CUP: Calories: 90 | Fat: 2.5g | Protein: 4g | Sodium: 510mg | Fiber: 3g | Carbohydrates: 14g

Roasted Corn Salad

Struggling to eat enough fresh vegetables? This tasty salad has generous helpings of corn and edamame, a high-protein soy bean.

INGREDIENTS | SERVES 6

2 cups fresh or frozen shelled edamame
½ cup fresh corn kernels
½ cup red peppers, diced
¼ cup red onions, diced
¼ cup green onions, diced
1 clove garlic, minced
¾ teaspoon salt
¼ teaspoon fresh ground black pepper
1 tablespoon olive oil
1 cup fresh tomatoes, chopped
¼ cup fresh basil leaves, chopped
1 tablespoon red wine vinegar
Juice of 1 lime

1. Preheat oven to 400°F.

2. Toss edamame, corn, peppers, onion, green onion, garlic, salt and pepper in bowl to coat.

3. Place on a sheet pan in a single layer on middle oven rack and roast until beans start to turn brown (approximately 10–12 minutes).

4. Place in the refrigerator to cool completely, then toss with remaining ingredients and serve chilled.

PER SERVING: Calories: 120 | Fat: 4.5g | Protein: 6g | Sodium: 310mg | Fiber: 4g | Carbohydrates: 13g

Fat-Free Fries

French fries are a diet killer, but these fat-free fries are a perfect solution to your craving for junk food.

INGREDIENTS | SERVES 2

Butter-flavored nonfat cooking spray
2 large Yukon gold potatoes, cut thin into fries
2 egg whites, beaten
Salt and pepper, to taste
Toasted garlic powder
Ground red chili flakes
Fresh minced chives

1. Thoroughly spray nonstick baking sheet with butter-flavored cooking spray.

2. Coat potatoes in egg whites and lay out single layer on sheet pan.

3. Sprinkle with salt and pepper, garlic powder, and chili flakes.

4. Bake at 350°F for 20 minutes, adding chives when almost done.

PER SERVING: Calories: 260 | Fat: 0g | Protein: 11g | Sodium: 75mg | Fiber: 4g | Carbohydrates: 53g

Asian Green Beans

Love Szechwan green beans but hate the fact that they are tossed in oil and finished with lots of salt? Try these beans!

INGREDIENTS | SERVES 4

1 pound fresh green beans
3 tablespoons canola oil
1 tablespoon minced ginger
1 tablespoon minced garlic
¼ cup low-sodium soy sauce
2 tablespoons hot garlic chili sauce
¼ cup rice wine vinegar
2 tablespoons teriyaki or Ponzu sauce
½ teaspoon sesame oil
1 teaspoon fresh chopped cilantro
1 tablespoon toasted peanuts, for garnish

1. Blanch green beans by bringing 4 cups of water to a boil in a saucepan. Boil green beans for 3 minutes, then run under very cold water; set aside.

2. Heat sauté pan and add oil, ginger, and garlic. Cook for 2 minutes.

3. Add remaining ingredients (except peanuts and green beans). Bring to a boil.

4. Add green beans and sauté over very high heat for 1 minute or until green beans are tender.

5. Garnish with peanuts and serve.

PER SERVING: Calories: 180 | Fat: 13g | Protein: 4g | Sodium: 890mg | Fiber: 4g | Carbohydrates: 13g

Marinated Greek Vegetable Salad and Bread

This salad is served on a thick French bread, making this salad filling enough to be an entire meal.

INGREDIENTS | SERVES 4

½ loaf French bread, cut into ½-inch chunks
¼ cup olive oil
¼ canola oil
⅛ cup lemon juice
Salt and pepper, to taste
1 English cucumber, cut in ¼-inch chunks
1 large tomato, cut in ½-inch chunks
1 small red onion, chopped
½ yellow squash, cut in half moons
½ cup black or Kalamata olives
1 tablespoon fresh dill, chopped
6 ounces low-fat feta cheese, crumbled
2 teaspoons chili oil

1. Lightly toast bread in oven to light brown.

2. In a large bowl, combine olive oil, canola oil, lemon juice, salt and pepper, cucumber, tomatoes, onion, squash, and olives. Toss to combine.

3. Finish with fresh dill, feta, and chili oil.

PER SERVING: Calories: 480 | Fat: 38g | Protein: 13g | Sodium: 950mg | Fiber: 3g | Carbohydrates: 25g

Trail Mix

Most trail mix has chocolate and other ingredients you may be trying to avoid. This version is filling, making a small serving go a long way.

INGREDIENTS | YIELDS 2½ QUARTS; SERVING SIZE ¼ CUP

2 cups fat-free or low-fat granola

¾ cup pecans

¾ cup almonds

1 cup flaked unsweetened coconut

½ cup seeded sunflower seeds

1 teaspoon cinnamon

1 teaspoon salt

1 cup sweet condensed milk

¼ cup canola oil

1 cup dried apple chips

½ cup raisins

½ cup dried cherries

½ cup dried blueberries

½ cup apricots

1. Preheat oven to 350°F.

2. Combine all ingredients except dried fruit. Place on sheet pan and toast for 1 hour, stirring often.

3. Remove from oven and add dried fruit.

4. Cool and store in airtight container.

PER SERVING: Calories: 140 | Fat: 8g | Protein: 3g | Sodium: 85mg | Fiber: 2g | Carbohydrates: 17g

An Ounce of Prevention

This recipe is more calorie-dense than most of the recipes in this book, but for a good reason. Keep a stash of this trail mix in your car or at your desk for times when you are hungry but your only options are fast food or something out of the vending machine. A small handful will energize you with protein and curb your hunger until you can have a proper meal.

Refried Beans with Baked Tortilla or Pita Chips

Fat-free refried beans make this dish a protein powerhouse without added fat.

INGREDIENTS | SERVES 6

1 tablespoon canola oil

1 yellow onion, diced fine

2 cloves garlic, smashed

1 pound pinto beans

2 bay leaves

2 tablespoons cumin

½ teaspoon cayenne

1 tablespoon coriander

4 cups vegetable stock or water

6 slices turkey bacon, diced

1 bunch cilantro

1. Heat oil in large saucepan and cook onions and garlic until tender, approximately 4 minutes.

2. Add remaining ingredients and cover with stock by 2 inches.

3. Bring to a boil and then reduce to a covered simmer.

4. Cook for about 2 hours—checking and adding additional stock if needed until beans are tender.

5. Drain and remove bay leaves and bacon.

6. Add beans to food processor and blend, adding liquid to form consistency of mashed potatoes.

7. Adjust seasoning and serve with low-fat sour cream and baked tortilla/pita chips.

PER SERVING: Calories: 310 | Fat: 4.5g | Protein: 19g | Sodium: 60mg | Fiber: 15g | Carbohydrates: 50g

Green Pea Guacamole

Craving guacamole but dreading the calories? This "guacamole" is low in fat and surprisingly tasty for a dish that is avocado-free.

INGREDIENTS | SERVES 4

3 cups thawed frozen peas

2 tablespoons lime juice

1 cup red onion, chopped

2 teaspoons minced garlic

1 teaspoon cumin

Salt and fresh ground black pepper, to taste

⅛ teaspoon cayenne

½ jalapeño, seeded

½ bunch cilantro

1 tomato, diced

1. Combine and puree peas, lime juice, onion, garlic, cumin, salt, pepper, cayenne, and jalapeño in food processor.

2. Remove mixture from processor and add tomato and cilantro.

3. Serve cold and enjoy.

PER SERVING: Calories: 120 | Fat: 1g | Protein: 7g | Sodium: 125mg | Fiber: 6g | Carbohydrates: 22g

Serve with Salsa!

Serve this dip with regular salsa, and let your friends try to guess what kind of dip it is. They will never guess that it is made with green peas!

Toasted Orzo Pasta

Orzo has a nutty flavor when toasted, making it a heartier pasta that is more like a grain than a pasta. It is low in fat and soaks up the flavor of chicken stock.

INGREDIENTS | SERVES 6

½ pound orzo pasta

3 cups low-sodium chicken stock

¼ cup dry-packed sun-dried tomatoes, chopped

Salt and pepper, to taste

1 tablespoon dried thyme

1. Preheat oven to 350°F.

2. Place orzo on sheet pan in single layer and bake for 10 minutes until lightly browned.

3. In a large pot, bring stock to a boil. Add orzo, cook until tender.

4. Place sun-dried tomatoes in strainer and drain pasta into it.

5. Add salt and pepper and thyme and serve.

PER SERVING: Calories: 160 | Fat: 1.5g | Protein: 8g | Sodium: 85mg | Fiber: 2g | Carbohydrates: 31g

Roasted Vegetables

A great low-fat dish that can be used as a side dish, an ingredient in soups, or as a meal when combined with rice or protein.

INGREDIENTS | SERVES 4

1 large carrot, peeled and cut in thin diagonal cuts

1 medium red onion, peeled and cut into quarters

1 large zucchini, cut in 1-inch cubes

1 large yellow squash, cut into 1-inch cubes

½ small eggplant, cut in 1-inch cubes

1 red bell pepper, cut into cubes and seeded

¼ cup low-fat balsamic vinaigrette dressing

½ teaspoon ground black pepper

1 teaspoon dried Italian seasoning

1. Preheat oven to 375°F.

2. Toss vegetables in dressing, pepper, and Italian seasonings to coat.

3. Coat a sheet pan with nonstick cooking spray. Place vegetables in a single layer and roast for 12 to 15 minutes. Stir every 5 minutes while cooking.

PER SERVING: Calories: 90 | Fat: 1g | Protein: 4g | Sodium: 270mg | Fiber: 6g | Carbohydrates: 21g

Hoppin' John

This rice-and-bean dish is a traditional New Orleans favorite, eaten on New Year's Day for good luck.

INGREDIENTS | SERVES 8

½ cup turkey bacon, diced

6 ounces yellow onion, diced

1 medium red bell pepper, diced

2 stalks of celery, diced

4 cloves of garlic, minced

2 (12-ounce) cans black-eyed peas, drained

¾ cup low-sodium beef stock

⅛ teaspoon dried thyme

⅛ teaspoon red chili flakes

3 cups cooked brown rice

1 (14-ounce) can diced tomatoes

Diced green onions, for garnish

1. Combine turkey, onion, celery, peppers, and garlic in a skillet. Cook over medium heat until vegetables are tender, approximately 7 minutes.

2. Add black-eyed peas and beef stock to mixture; continue cooking until volume reduces by half, approximately 10 minutes.

3. Add thyme, chili flakes, rice, and tomatoes; cook until heated thoroughly, approximately 2 minutes. Garnish with green onions before serving.

PER SERVING: Calories: 230 | Fat: 5g | Protein: 11g | Sodium: 620mg | Fiber: 6g | Carbohydrates: 36g

CHAPTER 21

Soups

Hot and Sour Soup

A perennial Chinese take-out favorite, this soup is high in protein and low in fat, but still has all the flavor you enjoy from restaurants. This recipe makes enough to share with friends or freeze for later.

INGREDIENTS | SERVES 12

32 ounces low-sodium chicken stock

3 thin slices of ginger root, peeled

½ cup dried mushrooms

2 tablespoons low-sodium soy sauce

¼ cup rice wine vinegar

¼ teaspoon sesame oil

¼ teaspoon sugar

½ teaspoon white pepper

½ cup bamboo shoots, sliced into strips

½ cup water chestnuts, sliced into strips

½ cup fresh bean sprouts

½ cup firm tofu, diced into chunks

¼ cup carrots, shredded

¼ cup whole egg substitute

1. In a stockpot, bring chicken stock, ginger root, and mushrooms to a boil for 4 minutes.

2. Remove ginger root and add soy sauce, vinegar, sesame oil, sugar, pepper, bamboo shoots, water chestnuts, bean sprouts, tofu, and carrots and bring to a boil. Boil for 3–4 minutes.

3. Turn off heat and whisk egg substitute into soup. Serve while hot.

PER SERVING: Calories: 35 | Fat: 1g | Protein: 3g | Sodium: 120mg | Fiber: < 1g | Carbohydrates: 4g

Asian Broth

A super-flavorful broth to use as a base for a number of dishes.

INGREDIENTS | YIELDS 3 QUARTS; SERVING SIZE ¾ CUP

1 (49-ounce) can fat-free low-sodium chicken stock

½ cup Napa cabbage leaves, core removed and cut in thin strips

1 tablespoon low-sodium soy sauce

1 teaspoon garlic, minced

½ teaspoon dark sesame oil

1 ounce shiitake mushroom caps, dried

1. Combine all ingredients in a pan and bring to a simmer. Allow to simmer for 45 minutes until mushrooms are tender.

2. Strain for liquid diets or remove mushrooms, slice them, and return to broth.

PER SERVING: Calories: 5 | Fat: 0g | Protein: 1g | Sodium: 220mg | Fiber: 0g | Carbohydrates: 1g

Wonton Soup

Start with a batch of Asian Broth and let it simmer while you make the lean and tasty wontons that make this soup too tasty to resist.

INGREDIENTS | SERVES 8

1 recipe of Asian Broth (page 267)
2½ cups Napa cabbage leaves, core removed and chopped
1 pound lean ground pork
⅓ cup green onions, chopped
¼ teaspoon garlic powder
¼ teaspoon onion powder
½ teaspoon low-sodium soy sauce
½ cup water chestnuts, chopped
1 package wonton wrappers
3 tablespoons egg substitute

1. Preheat oven to 400°F.

2. Place broth and cabbage in a deep pan and bring to a simmer.

3. Combine pork, green onions, garlic powder, onion powder, soy sauce, egg substitute, water chestnuts, and 2 cups of cooked cabbage.

4. Mix well to combine and form into teaspoon-size balls.

5. Place balls on parchment-lined sheet pan and bake in oven for 5 minutes. Remove from oven and allow to cool.

6. Once cooled, place meatball in wonton wrapper; fold into a triangle and seal edges of the wrappers by moistening with water and pressing the edges together firmly.

7. Place in simmering broth and cook 3 to 4 minutes until they float. Serve immediately.

PER SERVING: Calories: 320 | Fat: 13g | Protein: 16g | Sodium: 370mg | Fiber: 2g | Carbohydrates: 34g

Spinach and Lentil Soup

Lentils are high enough in protein to replace meat in this vegetarian recipe.

INGREDIENTS | SERVES 6

1 cup dried lentils

5 cups low-sodium chicken or vegetable stock

1 teaspoon salt

2 tablespoons olive oil

2 cups onions, chopped

3 cloves garlic, smashed

¼ teaspoon cayenne

½ cup raw bulgur wheat

2 bay leaves

¼ cup parsley, chopped

2 cups tomatoes, chopped

¼ cup tomato paste

1 pinch dried rosemary

2 cups frozen spinach, chopped and drained

Salt and pepper, to taste

1. Rinse lentils in cold water. In a large pot, bring lentils, stock, and salt to a boil. Cover and reduce heat to a simmer for 40 minutes.

2. Heat large sauté pan over medium heat, then add oil, onions, garlic, cayenne, and wheat until lightly brown, then add in the bay leaves, parsley, tomatoes, tomato paste, and rosemary, and simmer for 15 minutes.

3. Combine stock and sautéed mixture (add more stock if needed), and add in the spinach right before serving. Season as desired with salt and pepper.

PER SERVING: Calories: 290 | Fat: 7g | Protein: 19g | Sodium: 510mg | Fiber: 10g | Carbohydrates: 45g

Roasted Vegetable Chili

This chili is vegetarian, but so filling that you'll never miss the meat.

INGREDIENTS | SERVES 8

1 pound eggplant, diced
1 pound yellow onion, diced
¾ pound tomatillos, diced
¾ pound zucchini, diced
¾ pound yellow squash, diced
1 jalapeño, seeded and diced
2 red peppers, diced
¼ pound carrots, diced
2 quarts low-sodium vegetable stock
10 ounces cooked red lentils
¼ head of cauliflower, chopped
1 teaspoon chili powder
1 teaspoon cumin
½ teaspoon salt
½ teaspoon freshly ground black pepper
½ teaspoon ground coriander

1. Preheat oven to 300°F.

2. Combine eggplant, onion, tomatillos, zucchini, squash, jalapeño, red peppers, and carrots onto a sheet pan and roast in oven for 15 minutes.

3. Place stock in a large pot. Add roasted vegetables to stock and simmer 5 minutes until tender. Add in lentils and spices.

4. Simmer for 5 minutes and serve.

PER SERVING: Calories: 220 | Fat: 1.5g | Protein: 13g | Sodium: 460mg | Fiber: 12g | Carbohydrates: 43g

Toppings

To make this chili look like a million bucks, top with a dollop of fat-free or low-fat sour cream, a sprinkling of low-fat cheese, and a few scallions. It will look like it came from a restaurant, but with the low-calorie, low-fat goodness of home.

Plantain and Corn Soup

Plantains are similar to bananas, only firmer and with more flavor. The sweetness of the plantains combines with the natural sweetness of corn to make a soup that is slightly sweet without added sugar.

INGREDIENTS | SERVES 4

1 tablespoon vegetable oil
1 medium onion, diced
1 clove garlic, smashed
1 medium plantain, sliced
1½ cups peeled diced tomatoes
½ cup frozen corn
½ teaspoon tarragon
1 quart low-sodium chicken stock
1 mild serrano chili pepper, seeded
1 pinch nutmeg
Salt and freshly ground black pepper
Fresh chopped parsley, for garnish

1. Heat large sauté pan over medium heat. When hot, add oil, onion, and garlic; cook until onions become translucent, approximately 8 minutes.

2. Add plantain, tomatoes, corn, and tarragon and cook for 5 minutes.

3. Add stock, chili pepper, nutmeg, salt, and pepper and simmer for 10 minutes.

4. Garnish with parsley and serve.

PER SERVING: Calories: 170 | Fat: 5g | Protein: 7g | Sodium: 115mg | Fiber: 3g | Carbohydrates: 29g

Bean and Barley Soup

On a cold night, this bean soup with barley and bacon will help warm you from the inside.

INGREDIENTS | SERVES 6

¾ cup dried navy or great northern beans, soaked
1 medium potato, peeled and diced
1 medium onion, peeled and diced
1 celery stalk, diced
1 small carrot, diced
1 bay leaf
2 sage leaves
1 sprig fresh rosemary
4 sprigs parsley
1 clove garlic, minced
½ cup pearl barley
¼ pound turkey bacon

1. In a large stock pot combine beans, potatoes, onions, celery, carrots, bay leaf, sage, rosemary, parsley, garlic, and 1 quart of water. Bring to a boil and simmer covered over low heat for 1 hour.

2. Rinse barley and place in sauté pan with bacon; cover with 1 quart of water and bring to a boil. Allow to boil for 5 minutes.

3. Add barley and any remaining water to soup mixture, and simmer 1 more hour, then adjust seasoning to taste and serve.

PER SERVING: Calories: 200 | Fat: 6g | Protein: 10g | Sodium: 450mg | Fiber: 6g | Carbohydrates: 27g

Broccoli Soup

This popular soup is made low in fat and low in calories without sacrificing flavor.

INGREDIENTS | SERVES 4

2 tablespoons canola oil

1 tablespoon butter

2 tablespoons garlic, minced

1 cup onion, diced

½ cup celery, diced

Salt and pepper, to taste

2 teaspoons fresh thyme, chopped

5 cups low-sodium vegetable stock

1½ pounds broccoli florets

2 cups packed baby spinach

2 teaspoons orange zest

1 cup low-fat buttermilk

2 teaspoons toasted pine nuts, for garnish

1 teaspoon nutmeg

1. Heat oil and butter in soup pot until very hot, approximately 2 minutes; add garlic and cook until light brown, approximately 2 minutes.

2. Add onion and celery; lower heat to medium. Add salt and pepper and cook until onions and celery are tender, approximately 10 minutes.

3. Add thyme, nutmeg, and vegetable stock; bring to a boil and simmer for 5 minutes. Add broccoli florets and cook 5 more minutes.

4. Add spinach, zest, and buttermilk, blending until smooth.

5. Adjust seasoning and garnish with pine nuts.

PER SERVING: Calories: 230 | Fat: 14g | Protein: 9g | Sodium: 480mg | Fiber: 6g | Carbohydrates: 21g

Bright Colors

This soup is a rich green color thanks to broccoli and spinach. Intensely colored vegetables—dark green spinach, bright red peppers, and orange carrots—are all rich in different types of vitamins and minerals. When possible, try to add a rainbow of colors to your diet, helping insure that you are getting a variety of nutrients.

Chickpea Tomato Soup

Chickpeas make this soup filling and rich in protein, while garlic, cumin, and turmeric make it flavorful.

INGREDIENTS | SERVES 4

¼ cup canola oil

2 cloves garlic, smashed

3 cups chickpeas, drained

1 small onion, chopped

2 teaspoons cumin

½ teaspoon ground cardamom

½ teaspoon chili powder

½ teaspoon ground ginger

½ teaspoon turmeric

Salt and pepper, to taste

2 cups low-sodium chicken stock

28 ounces chopped canned tomatoes

1 cup fat-free plain yogurt, for garnish

1. Place oil in heavy pan and heat. Add garlic and cook for 1 minute.

2. Blend chickpeas and onion in food processor and add to pot. Cook for 2–3 minutes.

3. Add cumin, cardamom, chili powder, ginger, turmeric, salt and pepper, and stock and simmer for 10 minutes.

4. Add tomatoes and simmer for 10 more minutes.

5. Season and garnish with a dollop of yogurt.

PER SERVING: Calories: 450 | Fat: 17g | Protein: 18g | Sodium: 940mg | Fiber: 11g | Carbohydrates: 60g

Sweet Corn Soup

If you love fresh sweet corn, this soup is for you. Filled with corn and smoked chicken with a hint of lime, this soup is best in the late summer when corn is in season.

INGREDIENTS | SERVES 4

10 ears fresh corn

1 tablespoon canola oil

1 yellow onion, chopped

½ cup smoked chicken meat or ½ cup diced turkey bacon (optional)

2 tablespoons cumin

1 teaspoon dry thyme

1 teaspoon dry mustard

2 tablespoons Worcestershire sauce

1 chipotle chili

2½ quarts vegetable stock

Juice of 1 lime

1. Brush corn with oil and grill. Roast until most of the kernels are brown, approximately 10 minutes. Cut kernels from ear and set aside.

2. In a large pan, sauté onion and chicken (or bacon) until tender, approximately 10 minutes.

3. Add cumin, thyme, mustard, and Worcestershire.

4. Add corn and chili with stock and simmer for 1 hour.

5. Using a blender, puree until smooth and strain into bowls. Season with lime juice. Garnish with fresh cilantro sprig.

PER SERVING: Calories: 310 | Fat: 8g | Protein: 13g | Sodium: 1,010mg | Fiber: 10g | Carbohydrates: 56g

Pumpkin Soup

Make this soup in the fall when ripe pumpkins are abundant. You can even keep the pumpkin seeds to make a tasty snack.

INGREDIENTS | SERVES 6

5 cups fresh pumpkin, peeled and diced

3 cloves garlic, smashed

2 medium yellow onions, peeled and chopped

2 bay leaves

¼ teaspoon marjoram

¼ teaspoon celery seed

1 cup canned chopped tomatoes

5 cups low-sodium vegetable or chicken stock

⅓ cup white wine

1 tablespoon honey

1 teaspoon cinnamon

Salt and pepper, to taste

½ cup skim milk

½ cup low-fat sour cream

1. In a large stock pot combine pumpkin, garlic, onions, bay leaves, marjoram, celery seed, tomatoes, stock, white wine, honey, cinnamon, and salt and pepper. Simmer until pumpkin is soft.

2. Remove bay leaves and place in blender. Blend for 30 seconds or until smooth.

3. Return to pot and add milk and sour cream; whisk to combine.

4. Adjust seasoning and serve.

PER SERVING: Calories: 150 | Fat: 4g | Protein: 8g | Sodium: 140mg | Fiber: 3g | Carbohydrates: 24g

No Canned Pumpkin!

Canned pumpkin doesn't taste nearly as good as fresh pumpkin, so avoid using it if at all possible. Canned pumpkin is often loaded with added sugar, which is another good reason not to use it!

Creamy White Chicken Chili

This creamy chili is satisfying and filling. High in protein, but low in fat, you'll be amazed at how much flavor a healthy soup can have.

INGREDIENTS | SERVES 10

1 pound boneless, skinless chicken breast, cubed

2 teaspoons garlic powder

1 large onion, chopped

2 tablespoons onion powder

1 tablespoon vegetable oil

3 (15-ounce) cans great northern beans

32 ounces low-fat chicken broth

½ cup chopped green chilies

1 teaspoon salt

1 teaspoon cumin

1 teaspoon oregano

¼ teaspoon cayenne pepper

½ teaspoon black pepper

16 ounces sour cream

1. In a large saucepan, sauté the chicken, garlic, onion, and onion powder in oil until chicken is just cooked through, approximately 7 minutes.

2. Add beans, broth, chilies, salt, cumin, oregano, cayenne, and pepper. Reduce heat, simmer uncovered for 30 minutes.

3. Remove from heat, stir in sour cream. Serve while hot.

PER SERVING: Calories: 350 | Fat: 12g | Protein: 27g | Sodium: 370mg | Fiber: 7g | Carbohydrates: 32g

Some Like It Hot!

This recipe can be as hot and spicy or as mild as you like. For a spicy version, double the cayenne and chilies, you can even add in some minced fresh jalapeños. If you prefer no heat, omit the cayenne and chilies and replace them with freshly chopped green and red peppers for color and added flavor.

Pumpkin Soup II

Pumpkin is high in fiber and vitamin C, along with a healthy dose of antioxidants. This autumn dish can also be made with acorn squash if fresh pumpkins are hard to find.

INGREDIENTS | SERVES 6

5 cups diced pumpkin

3 garlic cloves, diced

2 medium onions, chopped

2 bay leaves

¼ teaspoon marjoram

1 cup canned chopped tomatoes

5 cups low-sodium chicken or vegetable stock

⅓ cup white wine

1 tablespoon honey

1 teaspoon cinnamon

Salt and pepper, to taste

1 cup skim milk

½ cup low-fat sour cream

1. Combine all ingredients except skim milk and sour cream in large saucepan; simmer until pumpkin is soft, approximately 15 minutes.

2. Remove from heat. Remove bay leaves and place in blender. Blend for 30 seconds or until smooth.

3. Return mixture to pan. Whisk in skim milk and sour cream and serve.

PER SERVING: Calories: 140 | Fat: 4g | Protein: 8g | Sodium: 150mg | Fiber: 2g | Carbohydrates: 21g

Minestrone Soup

This traditional Italian soup is both hearty and flavorful, but very diet-friendly as it is low in calories, low in fat, and filled with vegetables.

INGREDIENTS | SERVES 6

3½ cups whole peeled tomatoes with juice

1½ cups chopped onion

1 clove garlic, minced

1½ cups low-sodium chicken stock

1 cup celery, chopped

1 cup frozen corn

1 cup chopped zucchini

1 cup canned red kidney beans

1 cup cabbage, chopped

1 teaspoon Italian seasoning

1. Chop tomatoes, then combine all ingredients in a large soup pot.

2. Bring to a steady simmer, then allow to simmer for 30 minutes or until vegetables are tender.

3. Adjust seasoning as desired and serve.

PER SERVING: Calories: 120 | Fat: 1g | Protein: 6g | Sodium: 350mg | Fiber: 6g | Carbohydrates: 25g

CHAPTER 22

Desserts and Snacks

Apple Crisp

This apple crisp filling goes beautifully with this crispy and crunchy recipe, but it can be used for other sweet treats as well.

INGREDIENTS | SERVES 12

Crust/Crumble

1 cup rolled oats
1 cup whole wheat flour
½ cup Grape Nuts cereal
1 teaspoon cinnamon
1 cup unsweetened apple juice

Filling

2 apples, sliced
½ cup raisins
1 cup unsweetened apple juice
2 teaspoons cinnamon
1 tablespoon lemon juice
2 teaspoons cornstarch

Choose Your Apple

If you prefer a tart apple crisp, try Granny Smith apples. For a softer texture try Fuji apples, and for a more intense apple flavor add Bromley apples. You can even try a blend of different types of apples, a little bit of each.

1. Preheat oven to 350°F.

2. Combine all crust/crumble ingredients and press half of mixture into the bottom of a 9-inch nonstick pan and bake for 5 minutes. Remove from oven and set aside.

3. Raise oven to 375°F.

4. In saucepan combine apples, raisins, apple juice, cinnamon, lemon juice, and cornstarch, and boil for 10 minutes.

5. Remove apples and raisins, placing them in the prepared crust, and reduce liquid until thick, approximately 5 minutes.

6. Pour liquid into crust and top with the remaining crumble mixture.

7. Bake for 30 minutes.

PER SERVING CRUST/CRUMBLES: Calories: 100 | Fat: 1g | Protein: 3g | Sodium: 30mg | Fiber: 3g | Carbohydrates: 20g

PER SERVING FILLING: Calories: 45 | Fat: 0g | Protein: 0g | Sodium: 0mg | Fiber: 1g | Carbohydrates: 11g

Low-Fat Tortilla Chips

Tortilla chips that come from a bag are usually deep fried, salted, and loaded with preservatives. Making your own puts you in control of how much fat and salt are in your chips.

INGREDIENTS | SERVES 1

2 corn or flour tortillas
Canola oil cooking spray
Juice from ½ of a fresh lime
1 teaspoon sea salt

Types of Tortillas

Look around your local grocery store and you may find a surprising array of tortillas. Whole wheat, sun-dried tomato, and spinach are among the many flavors now available.

1. Preheat oven to 350°F.

2. Cut tortillas into triangles and spray with enough oil to just moisten.

3. Lay out on a sheet pan in a single layer and bake until crisp, approximately 3 minutes. Tortillas will burn quickly so they should be closely monitored.

4. Sprinkle with lime juice and sea salt.

PER SERVING: Calories: 120 | Fat: 1.5g | Protein: 3g | Sodium: 2350mg | Fiber: 3g | Carbohydrates: 25g

Angel Food Cake

Angel food cake is typically loaded with sugar. This recipe uses Splenda instead of sugar, reducing the calorie content and making it safe for people who are prone to dumping syndrome.

INGREDIENTS | SERVES 16

12 egg whites, room temperature
¼ teaspoon kosher salt
1½ teaspoons cream of tartar
1 teaspoon almond extract
1 tablespoon orange zest
½ teaspoon lemon juice
1½ cups Splenda
1 cup cake flour

1. Preheat oven to 350°F.

2. Place eggs, salt, and cream of tartar in mixing bowl and whip on medium speed until frothy, then add almond extract, orange zest, and lemon juice and beat on high to soft peaks (about 3 minutes).

3. Slowly add Splenda and beat to stiff peaks (2 more minutes), then sift flour over whites and slowly fold in to combine.

4. Pour into a 10-inch nonstick angel food cake pan, and bake on middle rack for approximately 35 minutes.

5. Flip out onto a cooling rack to cool for about 1 hour.

PER SERVING: Calories: 50 | Fat: 0g | Protein: 3g | Sodium: 80mg | Fiber: 0g | Carbohydrates: 8g

Almost Fat-Free Cheesecake

You don't have to give up cheesecake to stay on your diet plan. Try this reduced-fat and reduced-sugar version, and you won't miss a thing.

INGREDIENTS | YIELDS 1 CAKE: 16 PORTIONS

1¾ cups fat free cookies, smashed into crumbs

¼ cup butter, melted

16 ounces fat-free or low-fat cream cheese

1 cup fat-free or low-fat sour cream

8 ounces low-fat or fat-free ricotta

2 cups stevia or Splenda

¾ cup egg substitute

2 teaspoons lemon zest

2 tablespoons lemon juice

1. Preheat oven to 325°F. Spray cheesecake pan (9-inch) with nonstick cooking spray.

2. Combine cookie crumbs and butter in a bowl then press into bottom and sides of pan. Bake crust 10 minutes then allow to cool.

3. Beat cream cheese, sour cream, and ricotta until fluffy, then add Splenda and egg a little bit at a time as you beat it in, scraping the sides of bowl often.

4. Add in juice and zest, stir to thoroughly combine, then pour into crust and bake for 60–75 minutes until light golden brown on top and slightly jiggly in the middle, yet firm. Do not over bake.

5. Allow to cool completely, then run knife around edges and cut into 16 portions and garnish with fresh berries.

PER SERVING: Calories: 130 | Fat: 4g | Protein: 8g | Sodium: 240mg | Fiber: 0g | Carbohydrates: 16g

Cherry Clafouti

No one will believe that this recipe is diet-friendly if you tell them. This recipe is rich, decadent, tart, and sweet all at the same time.

INGREDIENTS | SERVES 6

¼ cup + 2 teaspoons flour

½ teaspoon baking powder

¼ cup egg substitute

2 egg whites

⅓ cup Splenda

½ cup cherry or pomegranate juice

2½ cups frozen cherries, thawed and chopped

Zest of 1 orange

1. Preheat oven to 375°F.

2. Spray 8-inch baking dish with cooking spray.

3. In a small bowl, combine flour and baking powder.

4. In a separate bowl, combine egg substitute and egg whites; whip until frothy; add in Splenda, juice, and flour mixture; and mix until smooth and blended.

5. Fold in cherries and zest and ladle into baking dish; bake for 35–45 minutes until golden brown.

6. Allow to cool and serve with fat-free vanilla, frozen yogurt, or a dollop of low-fat whipped topping.

PER SERVING: Calories: 140 | Fat: 0.5g | Protein: 4g | Sodium: 80mg | Fiber: 2g | Carbohydrates: 30g

Low-Fat Bread Pudding

This low-fat bread pudding is so decadent that you will never notice that there is no sugar and very little fat.

INGREDIENTS | SERVES 8

1 large loaf of stale French bread, sliced
¾ cup golden raisins
½ cup egg substitute
¾ cup Splenda
3 cups skim milk
1 cup 2% milk
¼ cup butter, melted
1 tablespoon vanilla extract
Zest of 1 orange
1 teaspoon nutmeg

1. Preheat oven to 350°F.

2. Layer bread in a 4-quart baking dish that has been sprayed with nonstick cooking spray, and sprinkle with raisins.

3. Whisk together remaining ingredients and pour over bread, then allow to stand for 20 minutes, turning the bread over once.

4. Bake uncovered for 35–45 minutes and serve with fresh berries.

PER SERVING: Calories: 260 | Fat: 8g | Protein: 10g | Sodium: 330mg | Fiber: 2g | Carbohydrates: 37g

Fat-Free Granola

Avoid the high-fat store-bought version of granola by making your own at home.

INGREDIENTS | YIELDS 2½ QUARTS; SERVING SIZE ¼ CUP

7 cups old-fashioned rolled oats
2 cups wheat flakes (dry cereal)
2 tablespoons sunflower seeds
1 tablespoon chopped pecans
1 teaspoon cinnamon
¼ cup oat bran
¼ teaspoon ginger
1 cup molasses
⅓ cup honey
¼ cup raisins
¼ cup dried apples

1. Preheat oven to 350°F.

2. Mix together all ingredients except the raisins and apples on a sheet pan and bake until brown, stirring often.

3. Allow to cool slightly and add fruit. Enjoy.

PER SERVING: Calories: 120 | Fat: 1.5g | Protein: 3g | Sodium: 20mg | Fiber: 3g | Carbohydrates: 25g

Fat Free Tiramisu

Tiramisu doesn't have to be loaded with fat and calories to taste great. This version uses low-fat and fat-free dairy products, but retains the intense flavor of the full-fat version.

INGREDIENTS | SERVES 8

3 cups nonfat ricotta
1½ cups fat-free or low-fat cream cheese
1 cup Splenda
½ cup Marsala wine
2 teaspoons vanilla extract
3 cups fat-free or low-fat whipped topping
30 lady fingers (store bought)
1½ cups brewed coffee
2 tablespoons cocoa powder to garnish

Cocoa Powder

Cocoa powder is high in antioxidants, full of flavor, but completely sugar free. To make it tasty, you must add sweetness. Luckily, sweeteners like Splenda do the job nicely. If you love chocolate, you can use it to make your whipped dessert topping chocolate flavored.

1. Pulse ricotta in food processor until smooth.

2. Add cream cheese, Splenda, Marsala wine, and vanilla and mix to combine.

3. Fold in whipped topping ½ cup at a time.

4. Layer bottom of 13" × 9" dish with lady fingers. Brush with coffee to soak.

5. Cover lady fingers with ½ of the cheese mixture and smooth out.

6. Next layer remaining lady fingers over mixture and soak with coffee.

7. Add remaining cheese mixture and smooth top. Top with cocoa powder.

8. Cover and chill for at least 3 hours.

PER SERVING: Calories: 350 | Fat: 4.5g | Protein: 18g | Sodium: 410mg | Fiber: <1g | Carbohydrates: 46g

Grilled Fruit

With just a little bit of help fruit goes from a tasty snack to a decadent dessert.

INGREDIENTS | YIELD VARIES WITH FRUIT USED

2 tablespoons brown sugar
½ teaspoon chili powder
¼ teaspoon ground ginger
¼ teaspoon cinnamon
Pinch salt
2 cups fruit of choice (pineapple, peach, pear, apricot, apple), cut into thick slices and seeded/cored

1. Combine brown sugar, chili powder, ginger, cinnamon, and salt. Place cut side of fruit onto mixture to coat.

2. Place fruit on grill or nonstick pan at medium-high heat to allow sugars to caramelize, approximately 4 minutes.

3. Flip and cook for 2 more minutes. Flip and cook for an additional 2 minutes if fruit is not tender.

4. Serve with fat-free vanilla frozen yogurt.

PER SERVING: Calories: 260 | Fat: .5g | Protein: 2g | Sodium: 25mg | Fiber: 5g | Carbohydrates: 67g

Chocolate Pudding

This creamy pudding takes the guilt out of dessert! Indulge your sweet tooth without ruining your diet for the day or having a bad reaction to sugar.

INGREDIENTS | SERVES 3

1½ cups soy milk
3 tablespoons cornstarch
¼ teaspoon vanilla
¼ cup maple syrup
¼ cup cocoa powder

1. Combine ingredients in a saucepan over medium heat.

2. Stirring constantly, continue heating until mixture thickens.

3. Pour into a serving dish and chill to serve.

PER SERVING: Calories: 180 | Fat: 3.5g | Protein: 7g | Sodium: 70mg | Fiber: 4g | Carbohydrates: 35g

All Sugars Are Not Created Equal

Refined sugars can rapidly raise blood glucose levels and cause dumping syndrome. Less refined sugars, or "slow" sugars, are better tolerated, and while they have the same amount of calories as regular sugar, they are less likely to cause dumping syndrome.

Honey Granola

Granola is a fabulous food! It is high in protein, high in fiber, and very filling. Unfortunately, most granola that you can purchase is also very high in fat and sugar, so try this homemade version instead.

INGREDIENTS | YIELDS 8 CUPS; SERVING SIZE ¼ CUP

4 cups oatmeal

1 cup flaked or shredded unsweetened coconut

1 cup raw, hulled sunflower seeds

1 cup chopped walnuts (or nuts of your choice)

½ cup raw wheat germ

¼ cup flaxseed meal

¼ cup oil (canola or olive)

¼ cup pasteurized honey

1. Preheat oven to 350°F.

2. In a large bowl, mix oatmeal, coconut, sunflower seeds, walnuts, wheat germ, and flaxseed meal.

3. Combine oil and honey in microwaveable container and add a splash of water. Microwave for 15 seconds, then stir to combine thoroughly.

4. Pour honey mixture over dry ingredients in bowl, stir thoroughly to coat granola.

5. Spread mixture evenly on 2 cookie sheets and bake for 30 minutes or until granola reaches desired crunchiness. Use a spatula to stir granola every few minutes.

6. Allow to cool on cookie sheet, then store in an airtight container.

PER SERVING: Calories: 150 | Fat: 9g | Protein: 4g | Sodium: 0mg | Fiber: 3g | Carbohydrates: 15g

Italian Cheesecake

This recipe uses fat free granola (see Fat-Free Granola recipe page 282) for the crust rather than a butter-laden crust.

INGREDIENTS | YIELDS 1 CHEESECAKE, SERVES 9

1 cup fat free granola
¾ cup Splenda or sugar, divided use
1 teaspoon lemon zest
2 tablespoons light margarine
1 tablespoon Marsala wine or cooking sherry
Cooking spray
4 egg whites
1 pound light ricotta cheese
1 tablespoon flour
¼ cup sour cream
½ cup egg replacement
¼ cup evaporated skim milk
1 teaspoon vanilla

Dress Up Your Cheesecake!

Make your cheesecake a sensation by dressing it up with fresh fruit or a sauce made from all-fruit preserves! If you prefer a fruit sauce, combine equal amounts of preserves and orange juice and simmer. Allow to cool and drizzle over your cheesecake.

1. Preheat oven to 350°F.

2. Combine granola, 3 tablespoons of sugar, and lemon zest in food processor or blender. Grind to the consistency of corn meal, approximately 1 minute.

3. Add margarine and Marsala, and mix until a loose ball is formed.

4. Spray 9-inch cheesecake pan with cooking spray, press mixture into a crust on the bottom and sides of pan. Bake for 10 minutes.

5. Beat egg whites until they form stiff peaks. Set aside.

6. Combine ricotta, ½ cup of sugar, and flour, mix to combine. Set aside.

7. Combine sour cream, milk, egg replacement, and vanilla, mix to combine. Set aside.

8. Combine ricotta and sour cream mixtures. Slowly fold in egg whites, stirring just enough to combine.

9. Pour into pie shell. Bake for 55 minutes, then remove and allow to cool. Serve chilled.

PER SERVING: Calories: 200 | Fat: 11g | Protein: 10g | Sodium: 290mg | Fiber: <1g | Carbohydrates: 17g

Body Mass Index Chart

BMI	19	20	21	22	23	24	25	26	27	28	29	30	31	32	33	34	35	36	37	38	39	40	41	42	43	44	45	46	47	48	49	50	51	52	53	54
Height (inches)											**Body weight (pounds)**																									
58	91	96	100	105	110	115	119	124	129	134	138	143	148	153	158	162	167	172	177	181	186	191	196	201	205	210	215	220	224	229	234	239	244	248	253	258
59	94	99	104	109	114	119	124	128	133	138	143	148	153	158	163	168	173	178	183	188	193	198	203	208	212	217	222	227	232	237	242	247	252	257	262	267
60	97	102	107	112	118	123	128	133	138	143	148	153	158	163	168	174	179	184	189	194	199	204	209	215	220	225	230	235	240	245	250	255	261	266	271	276
61	100	106	111	116	122	127	132	137	143	148	153	158	164	169	174	180	185	190	195	201	206	211	217	222	227	232	238	243	248	254	259	264	269	275	280	285
62	104	109	115	120	126	131	136	142	147	153	158	164	169	175	180	186	191	196	202	207	213	218	224	229	235	240	246	251	256	262	267	273	278	284	289	295
63	107	113	118	124	130	135	141	146	152	158	163	169	175	180	186	191	197	203	208	214	220	225	231	237	242	248	254	259	265	270	278	282	287	293	299	304
64	110	116	122	128	134	140	145	151	157	163	169	174	180	186	192	197	204	209	215	221	227	232	238	244	250	256	262	267	273	279	285	291	296	302	308	314
65	114	120	126	132	138	144	150	156	162	168	174	180	186	192	198	204	210	216	222	228	234	240	246	252	258	264	270	276	282	288	294	300	306	312	318	324
66	118	124	130	136	142	148	155	161	167	173	179	186	192	198	204	210	216	223	229	235	241	247	253	260	266	272	278	284	291	297	303	309	315	322	328	334
67	121	127	134	140	146	153	159	166	172	178	185	191	198	204	211	217	223	230	236	242	249	255	261	268	274	280	287	293	299	306	312	319	325	331	338	344
68	125	131	138	144	151	158	164	171	177	184	190	197	203	210	216	223	230	236	243	249	256	262	269	276	282	289	295	302	308	315	322	328	335	341	348	354
69	128	135	142	149	155	162	169	176	182	189	196	203	209	216	223	230	236	243	250	257	263	270	277	284	291	297	304	311	318	324	331	338	345	351	358	365
70	132	139	146	153	160	167	174	181	188	195	202	209	216	222	229	236	243	250	257	264	271	278	285	292	299	306	313	320	327	334	341	348	355	362	369	376
71	136	143	150	157	165	172	179	186	193	200	208	215	222	229	236	243	250	257	265	272	279	286	293	301	308	315	322	329	338	343	351	358	365	372	379	386
72	140	147	154	162	169	177	184	191	199	206	213	221	228	235	242	250	258	265	272	279	287	294	302	309	316	324	331	338	346	353	361	368	375	383	390	397
73	144	151	159	166	174	182	189	197	204	212	219	227	235	242	250	257	265	272	280	288	295	302	310	318	325	333	340	348	355	363	371	378	386	393	401	408
74	148	155	163	171	179	186	194	202	210	218	225	233	241	249	256	264	272	280	287	295	303	311	319	326	334	342	350	358	365	373	381	389	396	404	412	420
75	152	160	168	176	184	192	200	208	216	224	232	240	248	256	264	272	279	287	295	303	311	319	327	335	343	351	359	367	375	383	391	399	407	415	423	431
76	156	164	172	180	189	197	205	213	221	230	238	246	254	263	271	279	287	295	304	312	320	328	336	344	353	361	369	377	385	394	402	410	418	426	435	443

Normal   **Overweight**   **Obese**   **Extreme Obesity**

Source: Adapted from Clinical Guidelines on the Identification, Evaluation, and Treatment of Overweight and Obesity in Adults: The Evidence Report.

APPENDIX B

Resources

Print Resources

Clean Eating Magazine (50 low-fat, low-calorie recipes each month). Monthly periodical. (Robert Kennedy Publishing Inc.)

Greeson, Janet. *It's Not What You're Eating, It's What's Eating You.* New York: Pocket Books, 1994.

Levine, Patt, and Michelle Bontempo-Saray. *Eating Well After Weight Loss Surgery.* New York: Da Capo Press, 2004.

Maar, Nancy T. *The Everything® Sugar-Free Cookbook.* Avon, MA: Adams Media, 2008.

Ornish, Dean, MD. *Eat More Weigh Less.* New York: Harper Collins, 1993.

Prevention Magazine. Monthly periodical. (Rodale, Inc.)

Rice, Pamela Hahn. *The Everything® Low-Salt Cookbook.* Avon, MA: Adams Media, 2004.

Shrik, Lynette Rhorer. *The Everything® Whole-Grain, High-Fiber Cookbook.* Avon, MA: Adams Media, 2008.

Woodruff, Sandra. *The Good Carb Cookbook: Secrets of Eating Low on the Glycemic Index.* New York: Avery Publishing Group, 2001.

Online Resources

Obesityhelp.com
Online support forum, categorized by type of surgery.
www.obesityhelp.com

LivingAfterWLS.com
Online support, recipes, and more.
www.livingafterwls.com

Plasticsurgery.about.com
Physician-reviewed information on plastic surgery after weight loss procedures.
www.plasticsurgery.about.com

Index

Accountability, 53
Alcohol, 10, 11, 82, 117
Anastomosis, 44
Anesthesia side effects, 28–29
Anger, 78–79
Apples
  about: peels, 185; types of, 278
  Apple and Rice Smoothie, 185
  Apple Crisp, 278
  Chunky Apple Sauce Muffins, 177
Avocado
  Avocado Dressing, 190
  Avocado Tofu Smoothie, 182
Baked sweets, 145
Baking, 137–38
Bananas, in smoothies, 181, 184, 185–86
Bands. See Restrictive procedures
BBQ. See Marinades, dressings, rubs, and
  sauces
Beans. See Legumes and beans
Beef, **220**
  about: tenderloin, 222
  Asian Flank Steak with Edamame and
    Soba, 226
  Beef (or Lamb) Stew with Apricots and
    Saffron, 221
  Beef Kabobs, 221
  Beefy Onion Belgian Stew, 244
  Mini Meat Loaf, 225
  Pizzaiola Steaks, 230
  Tequila Lime London Broil, 230
  Turkey Bacon-Wrapped Beef Tenderloin,
    222
Birth control, 14
Bleeding after surgery, 26
Blood clots (DVT), 27
Body image and self-esteem, 73–74, 170
Body mass index chart, 287
Boiling, 139
Braising, 140
Breads
  Chunky Apple Sauce Muffins, 177
  Marinated Greek Vegetable Salad and
    Bread, 261
  Pancakes, 176
Breathing difficulties, 27
Broccoli Soup, 272
Broiling, 138
Burritos, 224
Buttermilk Marinade, 191
Butter substitutes, 233, 255
Bypass (malabsorptive) surgery
  dumping syndrome after, 36–37
  excessive weight loss after, 45
  fat soluble vitamin deficiency after, 43–44

incisional hernias after, 45
kidney stones after, 41–42
long-term issues after, 41–46
malnutrition after, 42–43
osteoporosis after, 43
post-surgery considerations, 36–38
pregnancy after, 46
stenosis, strictures, and ulcers after, 44
tiny meals, pouch capacity and, 37–38
types and nature of, 32–33
Cabbage
  Cabbage Rolls with Tomato Sauce, 246
  Wonton Soup, 268
Cabbage Roll Sauce, 247
Calories. See Portion and calorie control
Candied food, 144
Change, coping with, 71–72. See also
  Emotional issues
Cheese
  about: to avoid, 145; cottage cheese, 180;
    fat-free, 257; guidelines for eating, 111–
    12; reducing fat in recipes, 180
  Alfredo Sauce, 253
  Almost Fat-Free Cheesecake, 280
  Baked Mac and Cheese, 256
  Berry Cheese Blintzes, 250
  Fat Free Tiramisu, 283
  Italian Cheesecake, 286
  Low-Fat, High-Flavor Quiche, 254
  Zucchini-Onion Quiche, 178
Cherry Clafouti, 281
Chewing food, 33–35
Chicken. See Poultry
Chinese Five-Spice Rub, 191
Chocolate Pudding, 284
Citrus
  marinades, etc. with. See Marinades,
    dressings, rubs, and sauces
  Orange Maple Smoothie, 184
Coconut
  about: coconut milk, 182
  Coconut Curry Sauce, 198
Comfort food, guilt-free, **241**–57
Complications and side effects, 61–62. See
  also Bypass (malabsorptive) surgery;
  Restrictive procedures
  anesthesia side effects, 28–29
  emergency signs after surgery, 26–28
  managing complications, 62
  pain, 29–30
  stress of surgery and, 30
Concentric pouch dilation, 40
Cooking after surgery, 136–49
  easy substitutions, 141–44
  equipment for, 146–49

ideal techniques, 137–41
measuring devices for, 148–49
portions, 149. See also Portion and calorie
  control
techniques to avoid, 144–46
Cooking sprays, 147–48
Corn
  Low-Fat Tortilla Chips, 279
  Plantain and Corn Soup, 271
  Roasted Corn Salad, 260
  Sweet Corn Soup, 273
Crusts, 146
Dairy, 111–12
Depression, 67–68
Desserts and snacks, **277**–86
  about: to avoid, 145; cocoa powder, 283;
    snacking, 115–16; snacking and plateaus,
    157
  Almost Fat-Free Cheesecake, 280
  Angel Food Cake, 279
  Apple Crisp, 278
  Berry Cheese Blintzes, 250
  Cherry Clafouti, 281
  Chocolate Pudding, 284
  Fat-Free Granola, 282
  Fat Free Tiramisu, 283
  Grilled Fruit, 284
  Honey Granola, 285
  Italian Cheesecake, 286
  Low-Fat Bread Pudding, 282
  Low-Fat Tortilla Chips, 279
Dressings. See Marinades, dressings, rubs, and
  sauces
Drinks. See Smoothies and drinks
Drugs, 81–82. See also Alcohol
Drugs, prescription. See Medications
Dumping syndrome after, 36–37
Eating, 108–22
  avoiding pain, 116
  changing tastes and, 65, 110
  clean, 109
  difficulty after surgery, 61
  food choices, 52, 110–14
  foods to avoid, 118, 119–20
  insufficient quantities, 156–57
  learning to cook healthy meals, 65–66
  listening to your body, 119
  nutritional considerations, 110–14
  planning for indulgences, 160
  portion and calorie control, 52, 64–65,
    115–17, 126, 134–35, 149, 157–58
  during recovery period, 19–20
  in restaurants, 120–22
  restrictions, 109
  snacking, 115–16